Advance Praise f
Sustaining the Dignity and Nobility of Medical Care and Dr. Simone:

"The role of an oncologist is a difficult one. Providing information on prognosis, stage and therapeutic options requires a continuing need for self-education and communication skills. In an increasing environment of complicated issues regarding re-imbursement and insurance issues today's oncologist spends an increasing amount of time and energy on billing, forms, and regulations.

However, patients and family still need the care and compassion they deserve. Dr. Simone is the voice that reminds us of the central responsibility of a true oncologist."
— **Paul A. Bunn, Jr, MD,** University of Colorado Cancer Center

"Two types of individuals graduate from medical school. Those who view medicine as an occupation and those who view medicine as a vocation. The former are called Doctors. The latter, Physicians. Joe Simone is the ultimate physician, who by example and by his writings, serves as one of the true giants of our field."
— **Patrick J. Loehrer, Sr, MD,** Indiana University Melvin and Bren Simon Cancer Center

"Dr. Simone provides unusual insights into what it means to be a physician."
— **James O. Armitage, MD,** University of Nebraska Medical Center

Published by Editorial Rx Press

Editorial Rx Press, Registered Office: P.O. Box 794,
Orange Park, FL 32067
www.editorialrxpress.com

First Editorial Rx Press Printing October 2007
10 9 8 7 6 5 4 3 2 1

Copyright © Joseph V. Simone, MD
All rights reserved

ISBN 978-0-9799274-0-9

Printed in the United States of America
Original cover and book layout design by Biographics

Without limiting the rights under copyright reserved above, no part of this publication may be reproduced, stored in or introduced into a retrieval system, or transmitted, in any form, or by any means (electronic, mechanical, photocopying, recording, or otherwise), without the prior written permission of both the copyright owner and the above publisher of the book.

SUSTAINING THE DIGNITY AND NOBILITY OF MEDICAL CARE

A Collection of Essays

By Joseph V. Simone, MD

CONTENTS

3 Foreword by Robert C. Young, MD
6 Acknowledgments
7 Introduction

Chapter 1

9 CARING FOR PATIENTS: PRACTICE AND POLICY

10 Telling Patients the Truth
14 Navigating the Medical System's Choppy Waters
17 Providers of Cancer Care – How Goes It?
22 Health Care Access, Quality and Economics in 1932: Ray Lyman Wilbur
26 Health Care Policy and the Poor
31 "Cancer Refugees"
34 Consumer-Directed Health Care
38 Patient Consent and Conflicts of Interest
41 Trying to Understand Medical Economics
45 Planning National Cancer Policy in Croatia
48 Ethics and Medical Economics: Rationing Care

Chapter 2

53 QUALITY OF CANCER CARE

54 The Quality Waves Are Coming
56 The Quality Waves Are Coming – What to Do?
59 Assessing the Quality of Cancer Care at the State Level
62 Policy Efforts to Improve the Quality of Cancer Care
66 The Many Faces of Quality Cancer Care
69 Pay for Performance
72 Pay for Performance—Dead or Alive
75 Slow Pace of Improvement in the Quality of Medical Care

Chapter 3

79 LIVING WITH DYING

80 Dying Patients and the Little Flame
83 Why Work in a Hospice?
86 Intimations of Mortality
90 A Poet Faces Cancer
92 My Mother
94 My Mother – Final Act
97 Mourning and Grieving For Chris
100 Death and Grieving Survivors
103 Albert and Samuel

CONTENTS

Chapter 4
105 BEING A DOCTOR

- 106 The Rise and Fall of Trust in the Medical Profession
- 110 Oncologists Who Make Me Proud to Be One
- 114 "Concierge Medicine" and Other Trends
- 118 Concierge Medicine Revisited
- 120 Doc-in-a-Drugstore?
- 123 A Doctor's Values from His Father
- 125 Making an Oncologist ~ the Chicago Cubs Factor
- 128 Walker Percy
- 132 William Carlos Williams
- 136 Influential Books
- 140 Protecting Patients from Us
- 142 Dealing with Change in Oncology
- 145 Retirement Adventures
- 148 On Giving Advice and Offering Some

Chapter 5
151 MEDICAL ETHICS AND VALUES

- 152 Conflicts of Interest in Medical Practice
- 156 "The Stonemason" on the Integrity and Sanctity of Work
- 159 Client Billing and Self-Referral
- 163 Are We Single Agents, Double Agents, or Free Agents?
- 165 Econo-Docs in Oncology
- 168 The Role of a Professional Society in Medical Ethics-1
- 171 The Role of a Professional Society in Medical Ethics-2
- 174 Oncology Professional Meetings: Too Big? Too Commercial?
- 178 Uncertainty and Ethics in Clinical Trials-1
- 181 Uncertainty and Ethics in Clinical Trials-2

Chapter 6
183 LEADERSHIP IN MEDICINE

- 184 What Makes a Great Leader?
- 187 Leadership of the Food and Drug Administration
- 190 The Five Deadly Sins of Leadership
- 194 Pruning the Rosebush
- 197 Understanding Effective Leadership

Chapter 7
201 CANCER RESEARCH

- 202 Childhood Cancer Research: A Victim of Success and Bureaucracy
- 204 Childhood Cancer: An Orphan of New Drug Development
- 206 NCI's Cancer Centers Program – A Jewel Needing Polish
- 211 The Transformation of Cancer Research
- 214 A Cautionary Tale

- 219 About the Author

Foreword
By Robert C. Young, MD

IT'S A SAD FACT that most of a physician's precious reading time is necessarily spent focused on the continued advances in science and medicine. To be sure, those subjects should play a central role in ensuring that doctors stay on the forefront of medicine so that their patients benefit from the latest medical advances. But the vast majority of the thousands of medical and scientific journals and the tens of thousands of books devoted to medicine rarely touch on many of the personal aspects of medicine that play such a pivotal role in what makes a good physician. Nor are these humane aspects of the practice of medicine a centerpiece of medical school or house staff training. Such topics as ethics in medicine, principled medical economics, and the characteristics of medical leadership are rarely the subject of articles in traditional medical journals. When they are, the articles tend to be summations of the collective behavior of many physicians rather than the personal beliefs and motivation behind individual physician behavior.

That's what's so refreshing and satisfying about the collection of essays in this remarkable and insightful text by Dr. Joseph Simone. Joe's rich tapestry of experience comes through in every section of the book. A son of immigrant parents and blessed with a remarkably warm family environment, Joe has been a consummate pediatrician; a clinical investigator and visionary who has transformed the care of pediatric cancer patients; an administrative leader of two of the country's finest cancer centers and an advisor to many others (Fox Chase included); and, more recently, a volunteer hospice physician.

This collection of essays originally appeared in *Oncology Times* but here has been reconfigured around important themes. Having personally read most, but not all, of these essays in their original form, they are more powerful and enriching when arranged in the present format. Particularly the two chapters on "Caring for Patients" and "Living with Dying" address some of the most important aspects of becoming a fine and principled physician. Most of these insights would never be found in the conventional medical literature or in a medical school classroom. However, reading them here, and, more importantly, thinking deeply about the messages will likely enrich the quality of one's own medical practice.

Joe doesn't pull any punches in many of these essays and one will doubtless not agree with everything said. Nevertheless, his criticisms of "econo-docs," medical commercialism, and self-referrals are blunt, well reasoned, and applicable to a broad range of medical specialties far beyond oncology. Running through these essays is the premise that the practice of medicine is a noble profession and that there should be dignity and nobility in medical care. But Joe is experienced, wise, and self-confident enough to point out that medicine is a human pursuit accompanied by all of the usual flaws and weaknesses inherent in human behavior. Doctors after all are just people like everyone else. His thesis is that we must honestly recognize and address our weaknesses or we will never achieve the level of quality medicine to which all of us aspire.

Many of the chapters contain important references that direct the readers to other literature which expands and enhances the subject of the essay. Access to references on health care expenditures, consumer-directed health care, and ensuring quality cancer care are valuable sources of hard-to-find information. The chapter on influential books highlights Sinclair Lewis, Paul DeKruif, and Sir William Osler; I would personally add the wonderful works of Lewis Thomas including "*The Youngest Science and Lives of a Cell.*"

Another important example of the significant niche filled by these essays is the chapter "Leadership in Medicine." Although many physicians end up in leadership positions, almost nothing has been written about the characteristics of good medical leaders. Joe has utilized insights from business management writers such as Peter Drucker, Jim Collins, and Bill George to craft a series of essays on effective medical leadership. His ideas on criteria for enhancing medical leadership as well as tools for benchmarking the quality of leaders are illuminating and applicable to a wide range of medical settings.

But in my view, his essays are most powerful and most deeply affecting when they use his own personal experiences to illustrate important facets of the dignity and nobility of medicine. His volunteer role at Our Lady of Perpetual Help Home, an Atlanta hospice, as well as the people who work there provide one of the most endearing stories of the power and goodness of the human spirit. One cannot read those essays without concluding that even with all our human frailties, there is an inherent good that can be cultivated and maximized in all of us.

My favorite of all of these many wonderful essays are the two in the Chapter "Living with Dying," which he devoted to his mother's death. In the marvelous book by Sherwin Nuland "*How We Die,*" Nuland addresses the myth of the "good death." He points out that the physical act of death is rarely dignified and more commonly is difficult, wrenching, and solitary. It is the "spiritual" death with dignity that should be attainable and a skilled and sensitive physician can play an important role in the successful outcome. The warm interplay between Joe's mother and the family members, his willingness to freely admit when he didn't have the answers, and the careful suspension of medical interventions no longer relevant is a masterpiece of how a physician should interact with a patient at the end of life. Reading these two essays in *Oncology Times* in my office, I wept. Not for the death of someone I did not know, but for the spiritual death with dignity possible through the support of a loving family, a caring son, and a consummate physician.

I have learned a lot about myself as a physician and as a person from reading Joe Simone's essays. I believe they have helped make me a better physician and a better person.

There is much in these pages that will enrich your life as a physician and make you recognize the dignity and nobility of medical care.

Please find the time in the press of your medical responsibilities to make room for this insightful volume.

Robert C. Young, MD
Chancellor, Fox Chase Cancer Center

Acknowledgments

Pat Simone, my dear wife of nearly 50 years, began encouraging me to write long before I did so. She deserves my infinite gratitude for her rock solid support, patience, and wisdom over the years as we moved together through the various iterations of my career.

Serena Stockwell, Editor of *Oncology Times*, gave me the opportunity and support to try a new career as an essayist, offering her invaluable expertise along the way to a novice.

Deborah Whippen, the editor and publisher of this book, is largely responsible for its publication. She edited and arranged the essays into an appropriate format, managed the artistic input for the layout and cover, and arranged for printing and marketing. She is also a joy to work with.

Introduction

I HAVE BEEN A PHYSICIAN FOR NEARLY 50 YEARS. I have cared for patients, conducted research in the laboratory and in the clinic, led medical programs, and served as a senior executive of medical institutions. My perspective of the practice of medicine today has been shaped by that experience, but also by the influence of my environment, family, mentors, and colleagues.

Medicine is a noble calling and it is a rare privilege to care for patients. I have always believed strongly that we who have that privilege also bear the responsibility for respecting the essential nobility of providing medical care. For a variety of reasons it is challenging today in what we call modern medicine to sustain that spirit of care and to put trust in the system of care.

Many of the challenges, which are as old as the practice of medicine, have to do with medical ethics and money. There is far more money at stake in the current medical marketplace than at any time in history and companies that make products used in medical care have enormous financial and political influence. Some of the challenges are the product of social changes such as the nearly infinite pool of medical information available on the internet and the difficulty of applying that information to a particular situation. Another challenge is a product of the implicit belief by the public that there is a medicine to fix anything. This often leads to greater difficulty in accepting that one's medical problem cannot be cured or in facing the prospect of one's death or the death of a loved one.

Physicians face a more hostile environment today than in the past. They must deal to a far greater degree with government regulations, mounds of paperwork, and the sometimes contentious influence of insurance companies. The increasing complexity of care, the rising expectations of patients, and the constant struggle to keep up with advances and changes in medicine add to that burden. Each takes time—a commodity now more valuable than money for most physicians

Americans have long believed that they received the best medical care in the world. By a wide variety of measures, that position is no longer defensible. In public health, for example, infant mortality and longevity are areas in which the United States lags. The cost of care and the large number of uninsured patients are enmeshed in a hodge-podge system of care that is really not a system at all. The quality of care, and here I speak of cancer care which I know best, also is disappointing. The serious error rates in hospitals are scandalously high. And the quality of the practice of medicine ranges from outstanding to acceptable to shameful.

Many of these issues are influenced by leadership, for good or ill. Leadership is often underrated in medicine as an influence on ethics, quality, and the nobility of care.

I address all these issues and others in this collection of essays originally written as part of an ongoing series for *Oncology Times*, a trade paper directed to cancer physicians and nurses. This collection is newly organized according to the themes of what is most important and also most challenging in modern medicine today. These essays are my attempt to help sustain the noble spirit of the medical profession and its privilege of caring for patients.

Joseph V. Simone, MD
October 2007

Chapter 1
CARING FOR PATIENTS: PRACTICE AND POLICY

The interface between doctor and patient is the heart of medicine. It is influenced by the personalities, experience, knowledge, and trust of each. It is also influenced by forces outside the doctor's office, such as public policy, medical insurance, and medical economics. This complex relationship and its rewards and challenges led to these essays.

Telling Patients the Truth

AFTER READING THREE RECENT ARTICLES[1-3] published in the medical literature that deal with physicians' candor and "truthtelling," I was reminded of Pontius Pilate. In the Gospel of John, this Roman political leader was asked to decide whether Jesus should be executed. He believed Jesus had committed no capital crime. When he questioned Jesus about his actions, Jesus said that he was there to bear witness to the truth. Pilate famously responded "what is truth?" and ultimately agreed to have him executed to placate the angry and powerful crowd. Christian tradition vilifies him because he chose to sacrifice one powerless innocent man for political reasons. But there is a little bit of Pontius Pilate in all of us, as these articles attest.

Dr. Lindsay Rockwell, an oncology fellow, wrote a heartfelt essay in the *Journal of Clinical Oncology*[1] that laments the lack of "truthtelling" in oncology, particularly when it comes to the issue of death. She describes a young man with myelodysplastic syndrome and his father. The father complained to her that no one had told the family that the young man was dying, despite the short remissions and the inevitability of death. She is dismayed that death was not discussed and instead the discussions concerned additional therapy, none likely to succeed.

The essay was followed by a commentary by Timothy Moynihan and Linda Schapira.[4] They express concern at the damage that can be done by failing to communicate and that we often do not prepare our young physicians sufficiently in this art. But though they are in general agreement with the major points of the essay, they wonder whether the father was told but didn't hear the information, whether Dr. Rockwell was present for all discussions, or whether the father refused to give up and would not to face the reality of the impending death of his son. They even wonder, "Could it be that Rockwell is expressing her own grief as guilt for not speaking up when she saw the inevitable truth?"

What is truth?

Dr. Farr Curlin and colleagues wrote an article, "Religion, conscience, and controversial clinical practices," for the *New England Journal of Medicine*.[2] They conducted a random survey of physicians in all types of practice by mail and received 1,144 responses to questions devised to determine the physicians' judgments about their ethical rights and obligations when patients request a legal medical procedure to which the physician objects for ethical or religious reasons. Examples are abortion for failed contraception, giving terminal sedation to dying patients, and prescribing birth control to adolescents without parental consent. (The authors report that 52% of all respondents had ethical or religious objections to abortion for failed contraception.)

Most physicians responded that all doctors have an obligation to present all options (86%), that it is ethically permissible for doctors to explain to patients their moral objections (63%), but that they should then refer patients to another physician that has no objection to the requested procedure (71%). The authors then estimated the number of patients affected by the minority, if generalized to the entire population. They conclude that 40 to 100 million Americans have physicians that feel no obligation to present all options or who would not explain that they have moral or religious objections to the procedure and feel no obligation to refer them to a more agreeable physician.

Without questioning the sincerity and conviction of the respondents, we may ask who is more truthful, a physician who believes on ethical grounds that abortion for failed contraception is always wrong and doing anything to abet the procedure is also wrong, or the physician who believes abortion is wrong, but also holds that he cannot impose his views on patients so helps them find a willing physician? One could argue that the first is more truthful to his convictions and the second more truthful with the patient. One could also argue that the physician's first obligation is to the patient's well being, so he must help the patient obtain the procedure she desires, even though he thinks it wrong. The counterargument is that if he believes abortion in this case is murder, that he has no choice but to avoid abetting the patient.

What is truth?
The third article by David Studdert and colleagues[3] takes an economic look at telling the truth in, "Disclosure of medical injury: An improbable risk management strategy." They asked whether full disclosure of adverse outcomes actually reduces the providers' liability exposure, as some believe. They tested this theory by modeling the litigation consequences of disclosure. They compiled data on the historical frequency of litigation when the patient suffers a severe medical injury, both when due to negligence and when not. To obtain an estimate of the net impact of litigation, the authors polled 78 experts in patient safety, risk management, malpractice liability insurance, and plaintiff litigation, including lawyers on both sides. They defined serious injury as that which leaves the patient with a permanent disability or with a temporary disability that is very severe while it lasts.

They concluded from their study that, among patients whose severe injury was due to negligence, full disclosure would deter 32% of patients from suing and would prompt claims by 31% of those who would not otherwise have sued. Among patients whose injury was not due to negligence, disclosure would deter 57% of those who would have sued and prompt 17% of those who would not have sued. Overall, the experts predicted that there was a 5% chance that the volume of claims would decline or remain the same and a 95% chance that they would increase; the predicted outcome of compensation cost was the same, a 6% chance of declining and a 94% chance of increasing.

The authors make a key point: about 80% of all serious injuries due to negligence never trigger litigation. Thus, there is a huge reservoir of unlitigated injuries meaning a small shift in that group could have much greater financial repercussions for doctors, hospitals, and insurers than the deterrence from suing of an equal percentage of patients. Though the authors predict that full disclosure would cause an expansion of litigation and monetary consequences of potentially great magnitude, they do not say, "don't tell the patient if not forced to." The main audience of the report is policy makers, cautioning them to consider the consequences of full disclosure policies. They point out the broad consensus that disclosure of unanticipated outcomes is desirable because, as in other industries such as aviation, openness about error is critical to development of effective prevention. They continue, "there are also compelling ethical reasons for telling patients the truth about all aspects of their care."

So what will policy makers in government, the private health industry, and medical practices do? A cynic will say they will continue to follow traditional risk management procedures, which does not include full disclosure, to contain litigation costs and overall health costs. The optimist will say they will do the right thing, full disclosure, so errors may be addressed and corrected and improve the quality of care.

What is truth?

I am confident that every reader has opinions about each of these circumstances and I am equally confident that the most of those opinions are strongly held. But as is true for discussions of politics and religion, such case studies as those presented here often don't allow room for subtleties on any side for fear of taking a step onto a slippery slope that endangers a bedrock principle. One may hold a bedrock principle, but the specific circumstances tend to be messy and influenced by the many complexities of day-to-day living and by our own internal conflicts. We each have a moral/ethical compass formed by our parents, culture, education, and religious faith, or lack of it. However, these positions are not immutable; they can be modified by preachers, scientists, literature, travel, and other external influences, as well as by experience and the greater wisdom (we hope) that comes with age. But we still make "right" and "wrong" decisions.

So, what is truth? I don't have *the* answer, but I have an answer for myself. Truth in dealing with patients is based on transparency with humanity and charity that attempts to ease their burden. And for life in general, I believe my professor of moral theology had it right: for each individual a considerate, thoughtful, and well-informed conscience that takes all potential consequences seriously must be the final arbiter of right and wrong. My conscience always lets me know, at times reminding me even decades later, when I have acted against it.

10 April 2007

References

[1] Rockwell LE: Truthtelling. *J Clin Oncol* 25: 454-455, 2007

[2] Curlin FA, Lawrence RE, Chin MH, et al: Religion, conscience, and controversial clinical practices. *N Eng J Med* 356: 593-600, 2007

[3] Studdert DM, Mello MM, Gawande AA, et al: Disclosure of medical injury to patients: An improbable risk management strategy. *Health Aff* 26: 215-226, 2007

Navigating the Medical System's Choppy Waters

YOU ARE AN ONCOLOGIST. Your mother makes a routine visit to her internist who finds a lump in her breast that looks like cancer on the mammogram. What do you do? If you are smart, you do not take direct responsibility for her care. But you become involved.

You discuss the situation with her doctor and agree on which surgeon should see her and obtain the biopsy. You explain the situation to your mother and talk to the surgeon. The biopsy is positive and the surgeon recommends a mastectomy, though lumpectomy with adjuvant therapy is mentioned as another option. You explain the pros and cons of the options to your mother in more detail.

She chooses lumpectomy and node removal, which go off smoothly. The surgeon calls you to say the classical adenocarcinoma was completely resected with wide margins, but there were two positive axillary nodes. He says that he has explained this in detail to your mother, including the need for adjuvant therapy. You call your mother and discuss in more detail, answering her many questions concerning chemotherapy not addressed by the surgeon.

She is referred to a medical oncologist who meets your approval. After he sees her, you call him and he describes a plan for adjuvant chemotherapy that is to your satisfaction. You call your mother saying you agree with the planned chemotherapy, discuss more details, and help her plan for transportation, a companion during therapy, and for handling her normal duties. Your mother receives chemotherapy and tolerates it well; you talk to her before and after each course, offering her encouragement and support, and consult with her oncologist occasionally.

Following the chemotherapy, the oncologist recommends that she be referred for adjuvant radiation therapy. Your mother is wary so you call a radiation oncology colleague to get her view on the need for radiation. After your explanation of the advisability and potential consequences of the radiation, your mother decides to go ahead. Your mother completes the therapy without incident and continues to do well one year later with no lasting side effects.

The key medical feature of this story is that you helped your mother navigate The System of offices, institutions, and series of specialists. Her course was medically uncomplicated, but your mother was at times confused by the options or unclear as to exactly why a treatment was recommended. This process took a lot of your time and the physical outcome may or may not be any different than without your involvement. But it made things much easier for your mother; it gave her more clear information, more time for questions and answers, another view of the treatment options, and, perhaps most important, it gave her more confidence in the process and greater peace of mind.

Is this navigation of The System provided to patients who don't have a relative or friend in the business to help them? Too often, the answer is "No." Medical oncologists and office nurses sometimes, and pediatric oncologists more often, navigate for their patients' care. But many patients with cancer complain that: 1) "Different doctors are making different recommendations; they don't seem to have discussed my case." 2) "It seems clear in the office, but when I think of other questions at home, it is so hard to call in to clarify things." 3) "I was referred to a specialist doctor who didn't know my history," or "he had the facts wrong." 4) "My treatment was delayed for weeks because my records (or lab tests, pathology report, slides, x-rays) weren't sent (or received) by the specialist." 5) "There is so much information that I get confused, and my family and friends tell me even more to add to my confusion." Add to this the fear, anxiety, and disruption of family routine that always bedevils patients with cancer and it is easy, even for a good and well-meaning system, to add to the fear and anxiety.

A navigator helps a lot, so why is this service often not provided? That's easy: 1) It takes an enormous amount of time. 2) That time is not compensated by third-party payers. 3) Busy doctors and nurses usually assume that The System works efficiently and equally for all patients.

Navigators are not a new idea; among others, Dr. Harold Freeman successfully pioneered the use of navigators at Harlem Hospital many years ago. If navigators are such a good idea, who are they and how do we make them more available?

An oncology navigator should be knowledgeable about the diseases and treatments and should be comfortable negotiating through The System of care. The navigator must have the people skills needed to deal with medical, nursing, and administrative staffs, to provide clear information and comfort to patients, and to understand and respect the sensitivities of providers and patients. These options are not mutually exclusive and there may be others of which I am unaware.

Here are a few options to consider and my reactions to them:
- The best option is to get Medicare (and other third-party payers) to reimburse oncologists for providing well-defined navigation services. This is the first option, but a long shot in the current political environment.
- Train nurses for this role and seek reimbursement for their services. I like this one

because most nurses have the greater patience so useful in this role, reimbursement might be easier to negotiate with third-party payers, and hospitals and doctors offices might be more willing to chip in for the cost.
- Bring retired oncologists, surgeons, and pediatric oncologists into practices to provide the service either pro bono or for a modest, needs-based fee.
- Develop a pool of navigators from other disciplines, e.g., social workers or trained volunteers. Non-profit agencies like the American Cancer Society currently are testing such an approach using trained volunteers.

In short, if a navigator is good for our mothers, shouldn't we make this service available to all of our patients who need it?

10 November 2003

Providers of Cancer Care – How Goes It?

WE EACH HAVE PERSONAL VIEWS on the health of clinical oncology and often hear from prominent members of the cancer community on the issue. But we seldom see in print the views of those in the trenches. I have asked some private practice oncologists who I know, and who I judge to be thoughtful and open-minded, to provide their personal views for this essay. They represent practices of all sizes from all regions of the country. I suggested they use the "SWOT" format, though that was not required. While the SWOT analysis (strengths, weaknesses, opportunities and threats) has almost become a cliché due to its often mechanical application in strategic planning, it nonetheless provides a disciplined outline for assessment. I specified no particular topics, only their personal views of the current state of oncologists providing cancer care in the United States today.

Below are all the opinions offered, in no particular order within each category. Every opinion is included, though the wording sometimes is edited lightly to clarify or save space, and duplicates are listed only once.

Strengths
- Opportunities for personal growth and service to the community
- Doctors' general good will and willingness to collaborate and learn
- Enormous national resources
- There has been (up to now) enough money in the system to provide social services and do clinical research, both of which are money losers
- The most robust medical scientific community in the world
- Explosion of knowledge and technology, promising new drugs; the shift to targeted, relatively non-toxic therapy
- The silent revolution of the introduction of effective adjunctive therapies to improve the quality of life, like anti-emetics, potent biphosphonates, growth factors, and pain therapy regimens
- A health care system that emphasizes care of the individual patient

- Excellent methods of communication and information exchange among providers
- Streamlined delivery systems and infrastructure make up-to-date care widely available
- Strong national organizations and networks (American Society of Clinical Oncology, American Society of Hematology, National Comprehensive Cancer Network, etc.)

Weaknesses
- Too much money in the system leads to physician excesses and unreasonable expectations of patients, often avoiding or postponing difficult decisions
- The rising costs of cancer therapy are not sustainable, no matter how much they squeeze the docs
- Technological advances have increased the cost of care further straining the system
- Failure to come to grips with rationing health care (e.g., millions for separating conjoined twins while American children go without routine health care)
- Pharmaceutical companies [and the public] conspire to use the flashy new drug with the greatest financial impact, not the greatest medical impact
- Politicians have explicitly protected big pharmaceutical companies (in the Medicare Modernization Act!!) from competitive pricing; so they and the Centers for Medicare & Medicaid Services put the oncologist in charge of rationing care as prices skyrocket [it is unclear who the Medicare Modernization Act benefits, besides politicians in an election year and pharmaceutical companies]
- I hate having to monitor the percent of Medicare patients in my practice due to poor reimbursement
- Failure to take responsibility for the rising cost of treating patients with metastatic disease; embracing very expensive agents that provide statistically significant, but clinically marginal benefit and little, if any, survival benefit
- Limited use of computerized order entry (COE); oncologists give drugs with the narrowest therapeutic/toxic window and should be in the vanguard of office-based COE
- Ugly competitive practices by other oncologists in my town
- Can't get compassionate docs to join my practice
- Lack of any [national] system of care (read the Institute of Medicine report on the "Quality Chasm")
- Oncology is quintessentially a multidisciplinary specialty; far too few patients are seen in multidisciplinary clinics where shared decision-making occurs most naturally
- Many patients express grave fears that their multiple doctors are not communicating [efficiently], and, in fact, we are not!
- Most care is excellent, but there are major areas of poor-quality care, especially in chemotherapy and cancer surgery
- Treatments known to be ineffective are given far too often

- Too many treatments are not cost effective
- Regulatory hurdles, such as multiple Institutional Review Boards s for clinical research, are becoming suffocating; no evidence that the burdens of regulations like Joint Commission on Accreditation of Health Care Organizations, American College of Surgeons, Clinical Laboratory Improvement Amendments have made care safer
- Most of us are too damn busy; access to me is increasingly difficult as we add nurse practitioners (who do a great job), leading to complaints by some patients
- Public dissatisfaction with the process of care; complex data presented by hurried physicians is difficult to understand and retain
- We oncologists think we are entitled to special treatment (compensation), just because [of our station in life]; if someone starts looking at what we get paid, it won't stand up to the light of day – it just isn't right
- The newest generation of oncologists often act like hourly workers and not professionals; it is hard to make a case that you are special if you act like a soda jerk and walk out when your "shift" is over
- The high cost of drugs in the face of a large under- or uninsured population that is aging, leading to an ever larger number of patients
- Mountains of insurance company paperwork
- Large organizations cooperate on politics, compete on care delivery; end-of-life care and cost effective care must involve both community and academic practices
- Poor data on incidence and outcomes and almost no data on costs
- [Too] close association of cancer associations and research funding by the pharmaceutical industry
- Leaders in our field can be seduced by their privilege and lose sight of what really goes on day-to-day; they see themselves as special or different from "LMD [local MD] oncologists"

Opportunities
- There are enormous opportunities because the "system" is so broken, dysfunctional, and non-existent, e.g., a single electronic medical record that can communicate across all systems and platforms; this is one of many opportunities for the federal government
- Use current technology to see how well we are doing and improve care (e.g., the Quality Oncology Practice Initiative)
- Huge opportunity for applying newer treatments (if we can afford to do it and stay in business), to offer them to all who need them and not squander resources carelessly
- Better systems of collaboration between community and academic oncologists; many academic centers are creating more community oncologists but neglect development

of focused experts [to whom one can refer rare or difficult problems]
- A huge opportunity at improving the quality of care not only in medical oncology, but also surgical and radiation oncology, diagnostic imaging, and pathology; each has a major influence on the quality of care
- Improved methods of doctor-patient communication, decision support, and awareness
- Better models for management of patients with advanced cancer
- Move more toward skeptical, evidence-based oncology to take the high road in the quality, science, and delivery of care
- Better collaboration of national organizations with each other and with payers

Threats
- The piece-meal approach to fixing systemic problems, e.g., the Medicare Modernization Act results in serious unintended (but foreseeable) consequences for patients
- Growing expectations for unreasonably positive outcomes due to hyper-optimism and marketing
- Potential for an adversarial breakdown of relations between hospitals and doctors; with money exiting the system, physician purchases of CT and PET scanners, and radiation therapy equipment directly competes with hospitals
- Drug costs will price medical oncology therapy out of reach
- Ignoring rapidly rising drug costs for all, the inevitable increase in those who cannot afford care and the widening gap between those who can and cannot afford to pay for therapy
- Everyone else will police us and oncologists will no longer be the leaders of cancer care; there is a risk that "big brother" will have a greater interest in the bottom line than the quality of care–oncologists must create and maintain standards of care
- Continuously falling compensation may cause early retirements or curtailment of practices, leaving fewer, overly burdened practices; the public and Congress don't understand that at this rate we will end up with too few resources and providers to give care they expect

I close with two quotes that don't exactly fit in the categories above, but are illustrative examples of the depth of feeling among responding oncologists:

"These are exciting and frightening times for those of us in clinical oncology. The changes that are occurring have taken us by surprise because they have been so profound and have come so quickly, though none of us should be surprised by the changes."

"[The current situation is] not a pretty picture for someone who loves to apply exciting new technologies and feel the rewards of ... cancer care... What am I personally going to do? I am pleading with my partners to let me go to 70% practice time to try some new things for myself, like consulting. I'm 52 and due for a mid-life crisis! The rewards from clinical practice may be eclipsing and I'm too young to sit back and accept it all."

I thank the nine medical oncologists in community practice who wrote this essay: Al Casazza, Chris Desch[†], Peter Eisenberg, Dean Gesme, Denis Hammond, Russ Hoverman, Joe Jacobson, Mike Neuss, and Judy Schmidt. Their thoughtful words speak for themselves.

12 September 2004

[†]Deceased *(see "Mourning and Grieving for Chris" pp 97-99)*

Health Care Access, Quality, and Economics in 1932: Ray Lyman Wilbur

I RECEIVED A COPY of *The Milbank Quarterly* that celebrates the 100th anniversary of The Milbank Memorial Fund, which has supported individuals and organizations to address a wide range of topics in health and social policy. For its centenary issue, the *Quarterly*, published since 1923, has republished articles selected from its long history that were deemed to be interesting and important. Among the articles of special interest to me is the very first in the volume, by Dr. Ray Lyman Wilbur.[1]

Born in Iowa in 1875, Wilbur earned a B.A. and M.A. at Stanford University and then received his medical degree in 1899 from Cooper Medical College in San Francisco. He was to become one of the giants in medicine during the first half of the 20th century. He became the first dean of the Stanford Medical School in 1911 and was appointed president of the university in 1916. He continued to serve as president until 1943, during that tenure also serving as Secretary of the Interior under President Herbert Hoover. He then served as chancellor of the university until his death in 1949. He appeared on the cover of *Time Magazine* in 1927 and 1930.

Wilbur had been asked by the Milbank Memorial Fund to chair the Committee on the Costs of Medical Care; the Fund provided $1 million for the 5-year study (an amazingly large sum at that time). In March of 1932, Wilbur gave a 4th-year interim report entitled, *The Economics of Public Health and Medical Care*, at a dinner meeting of the Boards of Counsel of the Fund, and that report is reproduced in the anniversary issue of the Quarterly.[1] The report illustrates the thinking of medical leaders of the day and the health care problems they observed, especially the cost of medical care.

He describes the noble charge of his committee thus: "...a 5-year program of research in an endeavor to formulate a plan for providing adequate, scientific medical service to all the people, rich and poor, at a cost which can reasonably be met by them in their respective stations in life."

Wilbur then describes medical and economic circumstances of his day and the opportunity the work of the committee, if acted on, would offer. Some excerpts will provide a picture of the contemporary medical and social environment, and later, where he and the committee are headed.

In the European countries of his day, "Most of them have now adopted some form of governmentally-supervised sickness insurance, voluntary in a few instances and compulsory in the remainder, and the people now look to the central government to protect them against the hazards of sickness. In the United States, our history has been somewhat different."

He goes on to say that in America the individual States had largely retained control of education and medical service. He saw this as a unique opportunity, "With no central authority attempting to force uniformity of action on all parts of the country, we can try out a great variety of plans...We have no need ever of tying ourselves hard and fast to any one type of proposal." He did not foresee that the local governments' contribution to health care would largely remain the health departments, which dealt with issues such as water and food safety and immunizations, and the charity hospitals, like Bellevue in New York, Cook County in Chicago, and Charity Hospital in New Orleans. A more global approach would await Medicare and Medicaid in the 1960s, taken by the central government of which he was leery.

Wilbur then goes on to describe briefly the medical advances leading up to his day, mainly the control of smallpox, typhoid fever, yellow fever, and other infectious diseases through public health measures. He mentions the growth of research and infrastructure concerning the care of the sick, but not one advance in non-infectious diseases.

And then he gets into the heart of his presentation, beginning with shortcomings in the distribution, quality, and efficiency of care. "Measured by what is possible, however, in the light of present medical knowledge and technology, much remains undone. We *know* infinitely more than we *do* [italics mine]. Many of our people are untouched by the possibilities of preventive medicine. Some of them, we must admit, receive only second-rate care when ill and others are entirely without scientific care." Note that he says, "our people," a touching term of responsibility and solidarity.

"Some of our doctors are working today with the education given them thirty years ago. They are antiques that need re-polishing...Because medicine is so highly individualized it is, from the point of view of society, wasteful. Patients frequently spend much time going from one physician's office to another before they receive the necessary examinations or treatments...Sometimes the advice of different specialists conflicts and the patient doesn't realize that his greatest need is for a sane, well-trained general practitioner. Frequently examinations are repeated within a brief time. Over a period of years various physicians may have extensive records of a particular patient, records which duplicate each other in part, but none of which is complete. Sometimes, although there may be several physicians engaged on a single case, instruction regarding minor but important details is not given to the patient."

Does this sound familiar? I can almost hear patients, patient advocates, and some doctors cheering in the background today.

"The evidence is conclusive that our people do not yet receive all the benefits they could from modern medicine. For the rich and near-rich there is no real problem since they can command the very best science has to offer. The indigent and near-indigent usually, although by no means universally, are given a good grade of service by their local governments. Among the majority of the population, however, there are great islands of untreated or partially treated cases...Although it is a principle of far-reaching and, perhaps, of revolutionary significance, I think there are few who would deny that our ultimate objective should be to make these benefits available in full measure to all of the people."

He has clearly stated the problems, the goal, and the ideal, and then turns to the payment of medical costs. First, I offer some United States statistics from the late 1920s that will provide perspective. The average annual personal income in 1929 was about $750. The average annual personal income of a worker in a factory or mine was $1,000-1,600. The average annual farm income was $950. The average annual family income was about $2,500, usually with more than one earner per family. In New York, 32% of families had income below $2,000 annually in 1926. Physicians' income averaged $3,000-6,000, lower in the south, higher for specialists.

Wilbur describes research by his committee on medical costs done from a single year's records kept by 4,560 families in California and Vermont. Of these, 1,788 families had incomes below $2,000 annually and were classified as "low income." They found that 81% of families incurred medical costs of $100 or less, and he says, "we may assume, could pay their medical charges without serious hardship, but the remaining 19% must impair their living standards, draw on savings, or borrow money if they are to meet their expenses. Among the higher income groups, the situation is roughly similar."

Keep in mind that many families did not seek medical care at all, despite an apparent need; a survey done in New York at that time showed that 32% of families did not seek medical care for conditions more serious than colds or minor gastrointestinal disorders. Also, these data were collected just prior to the Great Depression, when average incomes dropped even lower. By the mid-1930s, my father was still earning less than $800 a year driving a taxi.

Wilbur responds to his own question, "Why is payment a problem," by citing two principal factors: the unpredictability of the timing and nature of illness, and "the uneven distribution of wealth in the United States and the apparent inability of a considerable number of people to do more than meet their current expenses." He goes on to say that public health is purchasable with fairly predictable positive results. "But to the *individual* [italics his], we must be much more guarded with our promises." With this uncertainty, it is psychologically difficult to save for future medical expenses, and even if one saved, there is no assurance that it will be enough; and for a large segment of the population, there is no money to save.

He next addresses how to pay for medical care. "Granted that good medicine is costly. I don't see how we [as a nation] can avoid paying the price. If we organize our talent for producing medical services economically and efficiently...we shall undoubtedly find out that the cost is not too great for our present society...The real nub of the economic problem is to determine whether the cost of good comprehensive medical care is within the reach of our people." He then remarks that if studies find that all but the indigent can pay the price, the only problem is finding suitable methods for collecting charges via insurance, industry, trade union, etc.

"On the other hand, if we find that there are substantial groups of people who, though not indigent, nevertheless have so little...that they cannot reasonably be expected to pay the cost of decent medical service...we face a different...and more vexing problem. Our sympathy, our sense of 'fair play,' and our desire for self-protection and self-preservation all unite in demanding that we reject emphatically any suggestion that these people should be given inferior service." He rejects dependence on charity to cover medical costs as distasteful to self-respecting people and too erratic and inadequate to meet such a large national problem.

The major concerns Wilbur addresses - the accessibility, quality, and cost of medical care - bedevil us yet today. Medicare, established 33 years after Wilbur's talk and despite its shortcomings, has partially addressed access and cost for many individuals. But viewed more globally, it is easy to see the irony that medical, social, and economic inefficiency may have become worse today. This is partly because there is so much more information to manage (much created by Medicare and other insurers) and so much more money at stake. And finally, the concerns he expresses about the uneven quality of care could have been written today, and have been.

While we justly marvel at the enormous technological advancement medicine has enjoyed since Wilbur's day, our satisfaction should be tempered with sadness. We have made far less progress in the access, quality, and universal affordability of medical care; and we are still swimming in an inefficient Babel of medical information at enormous cost. Wilbur's presentation of 74 years ago still has the power to inspire us with its insights, many still valid today. His humanity and integrity of purpose and his concern for those unable to help themselves shines just as bright today.

10 February 2006

Reference

[1] Wilbur RL: The economics of public health and medical care.1932. *Milbank Q*.83: 523-536, 2005

CARING FOR PATIENTS: PRACTICE AND POLICY

Health Care Policy and the Poor

NOT LONG AGO, WHILE IN A FOREIGN COUNTRY for a consulting job, I visited with the head of the state's health care system; he is a physician. His main interest was health care economics. We had a lively conversation that got around to care for the poor, which his state subsidizes. His position is best described as Social Darwinism, that is, people should receive as much health care as they can afford to pay for. So I asked, What if a poor cancer patient needed surgery, radiation, and chemotherapy to have chance of cure, but had only enough money (or insurance) for surgery? In effect, he responded, "Too bad. The state cannot afford to provide all the care everyone desires." I was stunned and pressed him, but he held firm. When I returned home, he had sent me an e-mail saying that he may have sounded heartless, but he had no tenable solution for health care for the poor, and by the way, he continued, what about the 40 million uninsured in the United States? He said he would like to hear what my solution would be. Here is my response, lightly edited.

Dear Sir:
I will start by saying that if I had a great solution to the problem of health care for the poor, I wouldn't be visiting your country but would be on my way to Stockholm for my Nobel Prize. This issue has bedeviled all economically developed countries, sooner or later, for the last 150 years. And the problem can be overwhelming in large parts of the world where there are simply no resources or there are corrupt governments that steal the country's assets for personal use. Since health care in your country started this dialogue, our discussion should be focused on the developed world.

I wish to be clear that I do not hold up the United States as a standard of uniformly high quality care or of having a rational approach to health care; we fail miserably in some areas. However, the 40 million uninsured should be explained. Studies have shown that about half are those temporarily uninsured for a few weeks or months, e.g., college students and the temporarily unemployed. So on average about 20 million, or about 7% of the population, are uninsured for an entire calendar year; some are self-employed, some are illegal immigrants, others choose not to have insurance, and many are poor and do not have the means. The most poignant are the working poor in low-paying jobs that offer little or no health insurance coverage and who do not qualify for government insurance; one of our failures.

Let me start with things I believe we probably will agree on.

1. No government or business has enough money to give people all the "free" medical care they desire.

2. Rationing of health care occurs in all systems, the instrument usually being one or more of the following: economic thresholds for the patient, government, or industry, depending on the source of payment; limitations of manpower or access to facilities; and poor quality of care that wastes resources, which includes overuse, underuse, and futile care.

3. Some out-of-pocket payment for care by the patient is desirable since many, if not most, have the money. The public, rich and poor, spends billions of dollars out-of-pocket on health care, such as over-the-counter pharmaceuticals, without ever seeing a physician or going to a clinic or hospital. We should keep in mind that much of this spending is discretionary and not covered by insurance and is an important part of the "health care dollar."

Now let me list some positions that I hold; I am not sure if we agree or disagree on them. These I pose mainly from the viewpoint of public policy rather than as a physician.

1. All patients should receive basic health care to assure that the state has a fundamentally healthy population. This is no different than the state, in its own economic interest, providing basic education for all. What is included in "basic health care" is a key issue and will be addressed later.

2. Some out-of-pocket payment for care by the patient is desirable, but should be graduated based on the gravity of the medical condition and the ability to pay. Even nominal payment of a few dollars for a doctor visit represents the patient's responsibility for the usage of care and has been shown to reduce frivolous usage. There are exceptions, however. For example, a patient with severe acute respiratory syndrome (SARS) or avian influenza must be treated regardless of the economics because he poses a major threat to public health. Or a destitute pregnant woman should receive prenatal care to reduce the chance of infant mortality or congenital disorders, regardless of ability to pay, because it is in the state's self interest to have healthy babies.

3. Our governments agonize over the cost of health care, but in the name of capitalism, close their eyes to some major causes of the high cost of care. For example, in both the United States and your country, prescription drugs account for a large part of health care costs, but our governments refrain from negotiating the same low wholesale prices obtained by large for-profit health systems. Fee-splitting, profiteering by physicians or hospitals, excessive testing, and "churning" patients are also a major drain. Health care cannot be treated as a commodity or as just another business that responds "normally" to market forces; it does not.

4. Poor quality of care costs more than high-quality care in the long run. A definition I favor is that high-quality care is medically justified, is provided humanely and with respect, safely, at the right time, in the right place, in the right amount, and without unnecessary pain and suffering. Futile chemotherapy for patients with terminal cancer, unnecessary surgery and diagnostic tests, medical errors, low rates of childhood immunization, and hospital-acquired infections are examples of poor care. They are like holes in the health care pocket draining resources from essential care because they use resources but are inefficient, dangerous, or wasteful. One cannot ignore the quality of care when considering the cost of care or access to care.

So what are the solutions to the burgeoning cost of care, the rationing of care, and care for the poor? There are no perfect solutions, but one at least can establish certain guiding principles. Here are a few I would espouse.

1. From a public policy point of view, the hierarchy of priorities for management of the health dollar starting with the most important should be: public health (e.g., water and food safety and sanitation); prevention (e.g., vaccines, prenatal care, smoking cessation, accident prevention); care of acute problems (e.g., injury, pneumonia, appendicitis); and care of chronic illnesses (e.g., cancer, diabetes, heart disease).

    This hierarchy proceeds from issues that can impact the most people or are most acute and the greatest threat to the state, to those that are less acute and occur more often among the elderly. In the first two, there are no patients, just relatively healthy citizens who the state serves to protect in its own interest. Much of the activity takes place without the knowledge of the citizen for the benefit of all, rich and poor alike in equal measure.

    In acute and chronic illnesses, the patient usually initiates the encounter with the health care system. When we talk about controlling costs, it is usually this patient-initiated care that we mean, and especially the management of chronic illness. The cost of a routine cholecystectomy is relatively cheap. On the other hand, a patient with diabetes, cancer, arteriosclerotic disease, Alzheimer's disease, or osteoarthritis faces years of therapy that may include surgery, radiation therapy, multiple medications and the management of complications and disability. I do not know the financial distribution of health care costs in your country, but in the United States it is these chronic illnesses, especially in the elderly, that consume the bulk of the money.

2. If the first guiding principle above is valid, then a health care system (public health is usually handled by a separate agency) should focus on the management and cost of chronic illnesses. A small savings in this category has a large impact on the overall health care budget. This is true regardless of the source of payment—government, private insurance, or cash directly from the patient.

3. Every patient should receive basic health care for his or her chronic illness, that is, what is known to be effective for controlling the disease and mitigating its effects. So all people with diabetes should have the means to control blood sugar and all children with leukemia should receive chemotherapy that has a 75% chance of curing the disease. Every person with debilitating arthritis should receive anti-inflammatory therapy and physical therapy. In other words, one can develop lists for each chronic illness of the components of basic health care that any humane system should cover.

4. The health care system should provide financial incentives for delivery of those basic services efficiently and cost-effectively, but also disincentives for care that is unproven or even wasteful, e.g., incentives for the use of generic drugs when available and older drugs that remain as effective as the newest, but more expensive version, and disincentives for excessive testing, futile care, fee-splitting and surgery of medically questionable value.

   The reimbursement systems in the United States and your country over-compensate those who perform technical procedures and under-compensate those who provide largely cognitive or supportive care. This rewards testing, procedures, and the resale of drugs to patients but not, for example, an internist who spends an hour helping a diabetic patient understand how to manage her blood sugar by diet, exercise, and insulin at home. Even a modest re-alignment of the financial incentives would, I believe, save money and improve the quality of care.

5. I would establish a quality of care program that helps develop management guidelines for common diseases that include recommended frequencies and type of necessary lab tests and radiography; these tend to reduce excessive radiography and laboratory testing. Guidelines should be developed by panels of physicians and nurses, including those with training or experience in health services research. The program should establish both medical and economic benchmarks and a mechanism for track-

ing outcomes in real time. Guidelines are just that, they leave some flexibility for judgment calls and are updated regularly.

6. Quality care does not mean that everyone requires immediate access to all non-urgent services or should expect amenities that have no impact on the quality or effectiveness of health care, such as hospital accoutrements.

7. It is my belief that health care system should ration care not by denying necessary care, but by eliminating waste, tracking effectiveness and outcomes and publishing the results, creating financial and other incentives for efficiency and disincentives for excessive testing, profiteering, and treatments that are unjustified by the evidence or other objective analysis.

In summary, I believe that all patients deserve basic health care as determined by scientific evidence and expert opinion; it is in the state's long-term interests. I believe that the quality of care should be tracked systematically and financial incentives established for efficient care based on evidence, and that the cost of care be reduced by cutting waste and excessive or unjustified testing and treatments. In that manner, all patients should be able to receive basic health care.

I recognize that this approach wouldn't be easy in practice, but if I were in your shoes, that would be my approach. I would be happy to receive any comments you may have.

Regards, Joe Simone, MD

I have not yet received a reply.

10 November 2005

CARING FOR PATIENTS: PRACTICE AND POLICY

"Cancer Refugees"

THE NATIONAL COST OF MEDICAL CARE and proposed solutions, largely through changes in public policy, is an important issue. But as a physician-oncologist, I believe that discussions about cancer care ultimately must begin and end with patients and what is effective, efficient, and prudent for them. We think we know, but sometimes our medical biases and economic interests get in the way. So an article in *The Wall Street Journal* by Peter Landers[1] on the intersection of policy and the patient is instructive.

The article was inspired by a speech made by Mr. Takashi Yamamoto to a session of the Japanese parliament with the Japanese prime minister present; Yamamoto is a member of parliament. He announced to his fellow members that he had cancer and then he proceeded to denounce the nation's standard of cancer care. He pointed out that cancer is the number one cause of death in Japan and that one in two Japanese will contract cancer and one in three will die of the disease. The article points out that the death rate from cancer in Japan has continued to climb since 1995, while it has slowly but steadily declined in the United States. In 2004 annual Japanese deaths per 100,000 from cancer far exceeded the number in this country.

Yamamoto continued: "However, the level of cancer care differs among regions and facilities. Even when there are treatments [available], people are being told they will never get better. These abandoned cancer refugees are roaming the Japanese archipelago. The health and labor ministry has set up an office for cancer policy...yet unfortunately it doesn't even have a grasp of...what level of care is being offered across the country."

Yamamoto then spoke against Japan's low-cost medical system (reimbursement rates are typically lower than in the United States). "If we cut reimbursement rates any more, we will accelerate the departure from the health care front line of medical professionals, who are already suffering from overwork out of a sense of mission. Take a look at the medical expenses on the receipt you receive at the hospital. The fees for expert services... how low they are. We need to have more flexibility in setting reimbursement rates, and we need to take a fresh look at expensive items such as foreign drugs and medical equipment. Some in the government are studying a further cut in reimbursements. This will lead to the destruction of health care. We must recognize that health care and nursing care contribute to the regional economies and create jobs."

So what was the response to this speech? Dr. Masaharu Nakajima, a surgeon who once treated patients with cancer and until recently was head of the Health Bureau of the Ministry of Health, Labor and Welfare, says Japan already offers excellent care. He said with the large national debt and corporations worried about higher taxes, Japan can't afford to throw money into treatments and training that offer little hope of significantly extending lifespans. "If we keep going like this, Japan is going to be crushed under medical expenses." Concerning the demand for more medical specialists, Nakajima responded, "America did too much of this and that's why their medical costs have grown."

The article then provides a framework for this Japanese debate. Health care spending in Japan is roughly one-half what it is in the United States and even lower than in Canada and Western European countries. However, Japan has the highest life expectancy in the world for women and the fourth highest for men, and it has one of the lowest infant mortality rates. Since introducing universal health insurance coverage around 1960, its policy has focused on providing a minimum standard of care for all. Japanese citizens and Japanese industry must pay monthly health insurance fees, but the central government sets the rules and reimbursement rates. However, unlike England, the doctors are in private practice, not government employees. Landers also points out that surgeons have an even greater role in determining the course of therapy than in the United States, including whether chemotherapy is given.

Another important cultural issue was illustrated thus: Shintaro Abe, a politician and the father of Japan's current Prime Minister, Shinzo Abe, was widely known to have cancer for two years before his death in 1991, but he was not told he had pancreatic cancer until two months before his death. Withholding the diagnosis is common in Japan.

Thus, the health care culture in Japan differs substantially from other economically strong countries from many angles. There is emerging change, mainly among patients. Patients with cancer are organizing and pushing for changes in accessibility to care and to effective new drugs. In May of 2005, 2,000 patients with cancer had their first meeting in Osaka. One of its organizers, Shoichi Miura, a physician who also has cancer, gave a speech recalling the rallying image of "cancer refugee" (gan nanmin). "While Japan has become economically prosperous, patients with cancer are in the same position as refugees who wander in search of food, water and *someone who can help* [italics mine]." He died 7 months later.

These efforts have borne some fruit. In April 2006, for the first time, 47 doctors who passed a rigorous exam were certified as oncologists qualified to administer chemotherapy. But the government continues to reduce reimbursement and increase co-payments by patients. Dr. Nakajima, the former health official, reflecting the government attitude, is opposed to raising reimbursements because corporate "executives want to keep costs down." He also says that a diligent surgeon who bones up on the latest literature can do just as good as a licensed oncologist.

Rather than react with smug superiority to the Japanese system, I was struck by how many of the issues are the same in our country. How do we balance the inherent conflict between patients' desire to obtain any care they wish and how to pay for such an open-ended system? How effective must therapy be to warrant financial support and who is to decide what therapy is effective? And how do we balance medically effective and cost-effective? How do we assure patients a high standard of quality cancer care regardless of where they live? How do we assure the same standard of care for the economically disadvantaged? What are the appropriate statistics for making policy decisions in cancer care? Do longevity and infant mortality always trump other measures?

More than academic discussions of medical economics, this story highlights the issues faced by patients and policy makers. Japan's approach makes economic sense and is supported by their excellent health statistics for longevity and infant mortality, and by their strong and highly competitive economy.

But the rapidly aging Japanese populace and the related increase in cancer mortality have raised awareness to several aspects of human nature that they must deal with. Cancer is the most feared disease in economically advanced countries, Japan included. Because of this fear, patients with cancer, compared with those with most other diseases, seem even more desperate for some hope to hang on to. This extraordinary fear has good and bad consequences. The good–patients often become very knowledgeable about their cancer, they are often willing to try new agents, and some become active in advocacy groups that raise awareness and funds for research and care. The bad–patients with cancer in their desperation are highly vulnerable to the "try anything" approach offered by well-meaning physicians (or by charlatans), even if the approach has no rational chance of making patients' remaining days better.

We in oncology have not systematically addressed these very human issues of fear and hope. On the one hand there is extraordinary fear and the vulnerability it creates, and on the other, how to offer reasonable hope based on intermediate goals when cure or remission is not in the cards. We need a better understanding and better tools for helping patients deal with their fears. We must not abandon patients once we know they will not respond to more cancer therapy. We must offer other kinds of hope without making the patients' remaining time a constant misery. We must always be *someone who can help."*

10 March 2007

Reference

[1] Landers P. Japan's 'cancer refugees' demand more options. *The Wall Street Journal*, January 11, 2007

CARING FOR PATIENTS: PRACTICE AND POLICY

Consumer-Directed Health Care

DEPENDING ON ONE'S POINT OF VIEW, consumer-directed health care (CDHC) is primarily an effort to: 1) control health care costs; 2) give patients more control of their health care; or 3) give patients "skin in the game," that is, the discretion and responsibility for spending dollars on the level of health care they wish or on non-health care expenses. In practice, CDHC involves enrollment in high-deductible health insurance plans which may or may not be associated with a personal health savings account (HSA) or a health reimbursement account (HRA). An HSA is a government-sponsored tax-advantaged savings account that may be used to pay for qualified medical expenses; it must be paired with a health plan of which the minimum deductible is $1,000 for individuals or $2,000 for families. An HRA is similar but it is owned by the employer and does not require enrollment in a high-deductible health plan (HDHP), usually defined as one with a deductible of at least $1,000.

The impact of such plans on the practice of medicine could be substantial, and not always for the better. Some providers fear a dramatic decrease in the use of products and services if such plans become the norm. I am a novice on this topic so a recent flurry of papers on the subject prompted this essay. Among them are two articles with some early data on the effects of CDHC by M.B. Buntin, et al. and by J.M. Yegian in *Health Affairs online*.[1,2] Also, several recent perspectives that appear in *Health Affairs online*[3-5] and in the *New England Journal of Medicine*[6] express a variety of opinions on CDHC.

The Buntin article[1] addresses the usage of high deductible insurance with personal health savings accounts, the cost and usage of care compared to traditional insurance, and the frequency of "favorable selection" in which healthier patients choose such health plans leaving less healthy patients in traditional plans.

Enrollment in HDHPs

The authors and others report that the enrollment in HDHPs is still quite low.[1,2] In data collected in 2005 only about 10% of privately insured non-elderly adults were enrolled and only about 10% of the enrollees had an HRA or HSA. About 20% of employers who offer health insurance also provide HDHPs and about 4% offered such a plan with an HSA or HRA option. But the authors state that demand is growing, with enrollment nearly tripling to 3.2 million since early 2005 and forecasts predicting enrollment of 15-30 million in 5-10 years. Also, 25% of firms that offer health insurance that do not include HDHPs say they plan to offer them in the next year.

Studies of favorable selection have so far found little difference in the average age of subscribers in HDHPs and traditional plans, but the former have higher incomes than the latter. Also, those in HDHPs seem to be in somewhat better health, based on data showing that usage of insurance was somewhat less *prior* to enrolling in an HDHP. So there appears to be a modest favorable selection for those enrolled in HDHPs.

Savings in Cost and Usage in HDHPs
The data show declines in the cost of care for enrollees in HDHPs, with high-end estimates of 4%-15% and low-end estimates of 2%-7%. However, the data is largely speculative and based on projections and must be viewed as provisional until better data are available. These studies provide varying results because they depend on factors such as the proportion of enrollees in a plan, favorable selection, and whether they also have HSAs or HRAs. Also, the baseline may be a moving target in response to these new plans, i.e., traditional plans may adapt to changes in the market.

Comparison of the usage of care is also difficult because of favorable selection, but the data that are available show a decrease in the usage of health care services in HDHPs. Two studies at a single employer showed lower usage of care for those enrolled in HDHPs than in traditional insurance. The cost of care, both out-of-pocket payments and plan spending, also was less.

Anecdotal reports in the trade literature report as typical savings for employers of 10% relative to expected trends with some reporting savings of 20-25%. However, some of these results refer only to employer savings and may be due to cost shifting to the employee.

Quality of Care in HDHPs
While studies have shown a decrease in the use of care by enrollees in HDHPs, reductions occurred both in care deemed efficacious and in services that are less effective. However, there was a clear reduction in the use of emergency services for less urgent problems and care was not reduced for services regarded as highly effective for non-poor children (no mention of the poor children). Add to these indecisive results and the difficulty of defining quality and the best one can say is that the effect on quality is mixed and far from settled.

Care of the Chronically Ill in HDHPs

A major concern for those in high deductible health plans is the coordination and cost of chronic care. Several case studies show a substantial increase in out-of-pocket medical costs for those with chronic illnesses, such as diabetes. Prior studies had demonstrated that increased patient cost-sharing reduced the use of both necessary and unnecessary care. However, more recent studies of tiered pharmacy benefit plans show that increased cost sharing leads to a reduction in the use of prescription drugs, including maintenance drugs for those with chronic illnesses such as diabetes and hypertension. (Studies of patients with cancer, if they exist, were not cited in these reports.)

The expert commentaries accompanying these papers demonstrate the breadth of opinion concerning consumer-directed health care. John Goodman is a strong proponent of such models of care because he believes that rationing of care is necessary and that patients are in the best position to choose the best use of the dollars in a system lacking infinite resources.[3] He also points out that patients may forego even necessary care because they live paycheck-to-paycheck and simply don't have the cash. That is why he believes HSAs are an essential part of high-deductible accounts. He concludes that the health plan must be well-designed to mitigate the omission of "necessary" therapy.

Marjorie Ginsburg, in her article entitled, "Rearranging the Deck Chairs," has a different view.[4] She believes CDHC "reflects health care providers' failure to deliver value and unrealistically assumes that consumers can make sound, cost-effective medical decisions." She goes on to say that the problem is not so much the overuse of services that are within the control of consumers (e.g., going to emergency rooms rather than urgent care centers), but the overuse of services that require physician authorization, such as diagnostic radiology or hospital admission. She believes patient preferences should always be taken into account, but such preferences cannot be a substitute for clinical indications and professional judgment, particularly for care that provides the best opportunity for long-term health.

In Tony Miller's article he advocates for consumer-directed care.[5] He was the co-founder and CEO of Divinity Health, one of the first consumer-directed health plans. He believes conventional health plans are part of the problem, pointing to deductible auto insurance as a better model. An essential aspect of the CDHP he founded was that it required an HRA. He believes decreasing or removing much of the current insurance regulations would allow development of even better financial models in the future.

M. Gregg Bloche reviews the history and arguments for and against CDHC and then points out the major problems with this approach: nearly all payers do not publicize their prices, there is a lack of information on providers' quality, and there is no means of assessing the efficacy of providers' tests and treatments.[6] "Research on efficacy has been limited by the resistance of drug and device makers and medical specialty societies, which fear that such information might reduce demand for their products and services. Health plans have the data to conduct more of this research but lack incentives to support it."

If these reports seem confusing and inconclusive, it's because they are. If the data are sparse and incomplete and experts seem to hold doctrinaire positions on the issue, how are we to understand the choices well enough to advise our patients? The many variables within and between plans make it difficult for patients to make choices that are in their best long-term interests.

Despite the paucity of data, the experts agree on one thing: CDHC is here to stay and it is growing rapidly. Employers are embracing this approach as a means of reducing their health care costs. The track record of our health care industry does not bode well for the development of consumer-directed health plans that are patient-friendly, that do not create disincentives for obtaining necessary care, and that provide transparent information on cost, quality, and efficacy. Unintended consequences of these plans, even if done with good intentions, could be disastrous for the health of many, particularly those in lower socio-economic groups.

25 December 2006

References

[1] Buntin MB, Damberg C, Haviland A, et al: Consumer-directed health care: Early evidence about effects on cost and quality. *Health Affairs* 25:w516-w530, 2006 (*web exclusive* www.healthaffairs.org)

[2] Yegian JM: Coordinated care in a 'consumer-driven' health system. *Health Affairs* 25: w516-w530, 2006 (*web exclusive* www.healthaffairs.org)

[3] Goodman JC: What is consumer-driven health care? *Health Affairs* 25:w540-w543, 2006 (*web exclusive* www.healthaffairs.org)

[4] Ginsburg PB: Rearranging the deck chairs. *Health Affairs* 26:w537-w539, 2006 (*web exclusive* www.healthaffairs.org)

[5] Miller T: Getting on the soapbox: Views of an innovator in consumer-directed care. *Health Affairs* 25:w549-w551, 2006 (*web exclusive* www.healthaffairs.org)

[6] Bloche MG. Consumer-directed health care. *N Eng J Med* 355:1756-1759, 2006

Patient Consent and Conflicts of Interest

THE ISSUE OF PATIENT CONSENT HAS INTRIGUED ME from my earliest days in oncology. The process always has seemed complex and even mysterious and certainly less straightforward than the legalistic consent forms may make it appear. Two articles in the *New England Journal of Medicine*[1,2] led me to re-examine my understanding of consent for medical care.

The first article by Campbell et al[1] examined the financial relationships between Institutional Review Board (IRB) members and industry in the IRBs of 100 academic institutions. They concluded that such relationships are common and that members sometimes participate in decisions about protocols sponsored by companies with which they have a financial relationship. They also found that about one-third of members never or rarely disclosed their relationship with industry. About one-third of members who had potential conflicts with a protocol under consideration and of those, one-fifth said they always voted on the protocol, one-tenth said they sometimes did, and about 15% said they did rarely or sometimes. The authors recommended that current policies and regulations be re-examined to assure that appropriate measures are in place to handle potential conflicts.

The second paper by Hampson, et al[2] interviewed 253 patients on cancer clinical trials to ask their attitude toward their doctors or cancer centers having financial relationships with the pharmaceutical industry. The result is what revived my interest in the whole consent process. More than 90% expressed little or no worry about such relationships and said they would have enrolled even if they had been informed of these relationships before entering the trial. A substantial minority said they wanted to be informed about the oversight system to protect against financial conflicts of interest, but I shall try to demonstrate that even this "after-the-fact" nod toward disclosure was probably more out of curiosity than worry that their doctor or cancer center would deliberately make potentially harmful decisions.

My own response to the first article was a lack of surprise at the presence of potential conflicts of interest among IRB members. Chemotherapy experts are asked to sit on

IRBs because of their expertise, and because of their expertise they are offered paid relationships by industry. The shoddy disclosure processes also don't surprise me, based on my own experience with IRBs. They are usually swamped with protocols and often struggle just to get the work done.

The second article[2] revived my long-held interest in the consent process, sharply underscored by the sheer coincidence that I was just then being asked to sign a consent form myself (for a minor surgical procedure, thank God). I called a colleague, Dr Steven Joffey from Dana-Farber Cancer Institute, who was a co-author of the article to discuss its meaning. I told him that I suspected the lack of concern expressed by the patients over financial conflicts of interest was not due to the specific issue at all, but that there was something else at work here; I just didn't know what it was or exactly how to articulate my idea. He was helpful and sent me a copy of another paper that he thought might help. He was right. The article, "An entrustment model of consent for surgical treatment of life-threatening illness: Perspectives of patients requiring esophagectomy," by M.F. McKneally and D.K. Martin[3] seemed to confirm my suspicions.

The purpose of the study was to describe the process of decision-making and consent to surgical treatment from the patients' perspective. I believe the results also apply to chemotherapy or transplantation for any life-threatening illness. The authors undertook multiple interviews with 36 patients who had recovered from esophagectomy for cancer. Their findings are summarized thus: "Instead of the accepted model of informed consent and shared decision-making, patients identified six concepts that describe their experience: 1) cultural belief in surgical care; 2) enhancement of trust through the referral process; 3) idealization of the specialist surgeon; 4) belief in expertise rather than medical information; 5) resignation to risks of treatment; and 6) acceptance of an expert recommendation as consent to treatment. These concepts were developed into a model of entrustment that unites the narratives of *all our patients* (italics mine)."

This jibed well with my own experience in over four decades of oncology practice and provided a plausible framework for what I have sensed but could not articulate. This would explain patients' lack of concern for financial conflicts of interest in the Hampson article.[2]

This also explains my personal reaction to the scary consent form for the day-hospital procedure I was to have, with words like "paraplegia, quadriplegia, cardiac arrest, or death." I questioned the nurse about that and she said, "Oh, we have to put that in because of the lawyers." I asked the surgeon about it and he said, "Oh, all that is from the anesthesiologists." My own problem was not life-threatening, but here I was doing exactly the same thing that the patients in the study did. In the end, I decided that I trusted the doctor and was in no position, despite having far more medical knowledge than the average patient, to try to manage all aspects of the process. Ultimately, a leap of faith was required and all six concepts described above applied in my decision-making (although "idealization of the specialist surgeon" is too strong for my taste).

The conclusions of the authors[3] also ring true and deserve more consideration. "There is a gap between accepted legal and ethical theories concerning consent and the patients' account of their experiences with surgical treatment of esophageal cancer. Although our findings should not be used to circumvent the ethical and legal requirements of the consent process and are limited to survivors of life-threatening disease, they support a careful reassessment of informed consent that includes the perspective of the patient."

In this age of patient empowerment, we often think that more information satisfies that requirement and that shared decision-making is based on the medical information that has been provided to the patient. This is true to an extent, but consent for medical care is a complex and different process in the patient than in the medical and legal systems. Understanding that process might make us better, more understanding care-givers and, as a bonus, might provide insight into how we might increase the number of patients who agree to participate in clinical trials.

10 February 2007

References

[1] Campbell EG, Weissman JS, Vogeli C, et al. Financial relationships between institutional review board members and industry. *N Eng J Med* 355:2321-2329, 2006

[2] Hampson LA, Agrawal M, Joffe S, et al. Patients' views on financial conflicts of interest in cancer research trials. *N Eng J Med* 355:2330-2337, 2006

[3] McKneally MF, Martin MF: An entrustment model of consent for surgical treatment of life-threatening illness: Perspectives of patients requiring esophagectomy. *J Thorac Cardiovasc Surg* 120: 264-269, 2000

Trying to Understand Medical Economics

MEDICAL ECONOMICS HAS BAFFLED ME FOR YEARS. I am an amateur trying to sort out the wealth of data and opinion offered by economists, health service researchers, and financially vested parties. All or part of the views of experts that I will relate below may be true. But I don't have a framework to know what is more important and deserving of greater attention, what is changeable (particularly by us), and what is more germane to high-quality care. First, I shall list several widely accepted descriptions of American health care.

1) Americans spend twice as much on health care as other developed countries, but the health of Americans lags behind those countries. This is blamed for the financial troubles of the American auto industry. 2) The health care industry is inefficient with a great deal of resources spent on administrative costs. 3) The lack of integration of government, private insurance, hospital, and provider services makes across-the-board systemic change almost impossible. 4) There are substantial regional variations in the quality and cost of care, with quality and cost sometimes inversely related.

Anna Bernasek in *The New York Times*[1] recaps the wide disparity in health care spending in American when compared to other developed countries. She then offers a solution: a single-payer system. She points out that this works well in Canada and some European countries and, as a bonus, the health statistics are better in those countries. She blames waste and inefficiency as a prime cause of the high health care costs in this country. She cites two studies that estimate that administrative costs alone account for 20% to 31% of health care costs and that much of that would be saved in a single-payer system. She says the stumbling block for a single-payer system is that most Americans don't believe in it. She believes it can work, but would take a great deal of time. Others, like Victor Fuchs at Stanford, are skeptical because of fundamental differences in the value system in the United States.

Eduardo Porter[2] writes that we are not getting our money's worth. He uses hospital expenditures for heart attack victims as a case in point. Such expenditures steadily rose from 1985-2002. However, while the 12-month survival rate rose in parallel with costs until 1995, since then it has remained the same. He believes one major reason is the regional disparities of care. The example used is that in the state of Iowa, 80% of heart attack victims receive a beta blocker within 24 hours compared to only 60% in Alabama or Georgia. This presumably leads to a higher 12-month mortality rate in the latter states and greater hospital costs.

Porter reports that this failure to adopt a well-proven, established intervention that saves lives and money has led Congress to decide to take some decisions out of the doctor's hands. The first step in this direction was the recently passed bill to offer a Medicare bonus to doctors who report on the quality of their care, such as prescribing beta blockers or aspirin for heart attack victims. (My own belief is that the carrot is often followed by a stick.)

The work of the eminent health economics group at Dartmouth, also reported in the article,[2] has shown in recent studies that there is no relationship between the amount spent on treating a patient and the quality and outcome of the care. For example, the cost of hospital care in the last two years of life for elderly, chronically ill patients dying in New York State hospitals was over $38,369, in Florida $29,604, and in Iowa $23,746. The same authors showed that hospitals in regions where the cost of care grew fastest had some of the worst records of using tried-and-true therapies and recorded the smallest gains in survival rates. Porter puts much of the blame on the fee-for-service system that rewards the use of aggressive, technologically driven therapy, too often providing little or no benefit.

Clayton Christensen, a professor at the Harvard Business School who has written books on innovation, was interviewed by William Holstein in *The New York Times*.[3] He laments the inefficiency of our health system and the relative inability of the medical industry to provide progressively more cost-efficient, convenient services compared to other industries. The industry excels at pushing "the leading edge of what's very difficult to do. But that's a very different dimension of performance improvement than the one that makes more people better off, and that is making it more affordable and accessible."

He believes substantive change requires disruptive technology instead of improvements in the existing system and uses examples from the computer world. Affordability and accessibility came not from building bigger mainframes, but from making the personal computer, in effect, by commoditizing mainframes. Michael Dell found he could assemble a computer in his dorm room, making personal computers a commodity. He believes much of medical care can be commoditized, as well. He bases this on the development of better diagnostic tools that enable a nurse, for example, to provide much of the routine care.

A final quote from Christensen: "The current health care system is divided into buckets. You have insurers, the employers who put up the money, the providers such as doctors and nurses, and hospitals. Because they exist as independent companies, they can each improve themselves, but they can't re-architect the system in the way that it needs to be changed."[3] He then cites Kaiser Permanente and Intermountain Health Care as rare health systems integrated across each of those pieces of the system. "They are far ahead of the rest of the world in bringing rules-based diagnosis and therapy in cost effective business models to their patients."

Victor Fuchs[4] would agree with many of the above statements, but not all, and he assigns a different level of importance to some. First, he says it is critical to understand that the high cost of health care in the United States has two very different aspects. The overall cost reported as a percentage of the Gross National Product depends on what people are willing to pay for health care *relative to cars or food or entertainment or other services*. By definition, all countries spend 100% of GNP and their citizens may choose to spend it differently. Americans, especially those with insurance, want ready access to specialists and new technology and, directly or not, they are willing to pay for it.

The other aspect of health care costs is the *rate of increase*. Studies show this is roughly the same in all developed countries and is driven by the introduction of new, expensive technologies. He believes this is where the best opportunity lies for reducing costs. He believes the United States needs a large, independent organization to assess the costs and effectiveness of new technologies and make that information readily available to physicians and other decision-makers. Such organizations have been established in Europe and had been particularly successful in England.

Fuchs debunks the idea that health care costs make United States industry less competitive.[4] He thinks this is based on the incorrect notion that employer-based insurance is paid out of profits, rather than being passed on to employees in lower wages. "The facts suggest just the opposite. Over the past 40 years, health insurance premiums have skyrocketed, but inflation-adjusted corporate profits per worker have doubled. On the other hand, inflation-adjusted wages of production and non-supervisory workers are lower now than they were 40 years ago." He believes arbitrary limits on spending for health care are unwarranted, just as they would be for education, food, or housing. It is more sensible to arrive at a system of health care delivery and finance that results in the same incremental value as other sectors of the economy. "That goal is reached when the last 1% of health care spending provides as much benefit as the same amount spent for [another social good], such as enrolling an additional 2 million children in Head Start or increasing the number of police officers by 50%."

Most observers agree that the current fee-for-service reimbursement system is bad, and not only from an economic point of view. It does not reward quality or efficiency or extensive discussions with patients and families. Instead, the incentives prompt more tests, more drugs, and expensive therapies of dubious benefit. Do we physicians bear any responsibility for this state of affairs? Can we just blame it all on "the system?" Or do we blame demanding patients with good insurance who "will just go elsewhere to get it?"

The "it" may be chemotherapy for widespread resistant cancer, or proton-beam therapy for general use, or the unnecessary colonoscopy that my physician recommended "and it won't cost you anything."

If we want to retain our independence and not have our practices "commoditized," we first must admit that we bear at least some responsibility for the current state of the economics of health care. Are we willing to lead or be led? Or are we hoping that any additional unpleasant changes occur after we retire?

25 February 2007

References

[1] Bernasek A: Health care problem? Check the American psyche. *The New York Times*, 31 December 2006

[2] Porter E: The more you pay, the better the care? Think twice. *The New York Times*, 17 December 2006

[3] Holstein W: Armchair M.B.A: For better care, work across lines. *The New York Times*, 31 December 2006

[4] Fuchs VR: Healch care expenditures reexamined. *Ann Int Med* 143: 76-78, 2005

CARING FOR PATIENTS: PRACTICE AND POLICY

Planning National Cancer Policy in Croatia

———⟫●⟪———

IS IT POSSIBLE TO PLAN, organize, and implement a successful national cancer plan...anywhere?

That was the first question that popped into my head when I received a call inviting me to participate in a workshop in Croatia that had that intention. Certainly it would be a fool's quest today in the United States. As one pundit said, the American health care system is neither a system nor does it promote health. Even the thought of trying to get a comprehensive plan through all the political and economic minefields gives me heartburn; and that is before considering implementation. But maybe, just maybe, a prosperous small country with a national health care system can.

I had never been to Croatia before and was not even sure of its exact location and size, or of much else about it. Croatia is a country of 4 million (80% of the Atlanta metro population) located due east across the Adriatic Sea from Italy. It is one of those small Balkan countries with a long history of always seeming to be part of larger political entities. For a long time before the First World War it was part of the Austro-Hungarian Empire—the architecture of the center of Zagreb, the capital, has a flavor of Vienna—and between the great wars the country was part of a Yugoslavia dominated by the Serbs. After World War Two, Josip Broz Tito took control of Yugoslavia until his death in 1980. Croatia became independent after the more recent Balkan conflicts in the 1990s.

Croatia calls itself a "transitional country," that is, not part of the third world and well on its way to a level of development qualitatively equivalent to other western European countries. It is stable and relatively prosperous and is due to enter the European Union in 2009. With its national health insurance, there is virtually universal access to health care.

With the help of the U.S. National Institutes of Health (NIH), especially the National Cancer Institute (NCI), and Croatian government ministers for science and health, oncology leaders convened a workshop with speakers from the United States and European Union as well as from Croatia and Slovenia, its similar neighbor at its north border. The goal of the workshop was to showcase a variety of approaches to the development of integrated oncology care and research systems and to end with a suggested plan suited specifically to Croatia. A similar catalyzing approach taken by the NIH with the Republic of Ireland has proved very successful.

The official goal of the meeting was to "determine opportunities and strategies for improving the treatment of cancer in Croatia." We met in Zagreb at the Regency Esplanade Hotel, which once served as a major stopover point for travelers on the Orient Express. Most of the attendees were Croatians from relevant medical disciplines, nurses and cancer survivors, as well as representatives of the government and its health and research agencies. Several Croatian-Americans participated, especially Drs. Steven Pavletic from the NCI, Branimir Sikic from Stanford, and Hedvig Hricak from Memorial Sloan-Kettering.

I am not sure what I expected to see and hear, but for me the meeting turned out to be a pleasant surprise. The atmosphere was permeated with a sense that we were participating in a rare opportunity for the country, one full of hope and optimism. And I learned a lot ~ about specific cancers from international experts, about technological advances in imaging, about organizing cancer care and research in Ireland and France and Holland, and about the growing patient and survivor advocacy movements in Europe and Croatia. I learned that smoking and lung cancer are big problems in Croatia, and also that they have a good cancer registry.

But most of all, I was greatly impressed by the determination of Croatian oncology leaders like Dr. Eduard Vrdoljak to improve the quality of cancer care and to develop excellent integrated programs for specific cancers that would stand up well with any in the world.

But the Croatians are realists. They know that their infrastructure must be improved, that they must find ways to train (at home and abroad) and retain their best and brightest young people. They know that the government must provide recurring and predictable support for these efforts to succeed. They know that the road ahead will be long and hard. But that does not dampen their enthusiasm and optimism one bit...after all, they are oncologists, and all oncologists are by nature optimists.

As of today, only one week after the end of the meeting, the written plan is just about finished, thanks to the leadership of Brandy Sikic and Steve Pavletic. Now it is up to the Croatians; we can help, but at the end of the day, the Croatian community must want this program passionately for it to be a success, they must be willing to persevere over the long term. If they succeed, even partially, they could be a model for other small countries that wish to do the same, and they will be able to advise others on what worked and what didn't.

I will watch the progress in Croatia with great interest, certainly because of having been there and gotten to know colleagues there. But I shall also watch carefully to see if the model they plan to follow succeeds. Organizing oncology care and research is difficult under the best of circumstances; success in Croatia could provide valuable lessons for smaller countries like Croatia.

Although Croatia faces a mountainous task, it was not lost on me that its scale and population resemble individual states in our country; we in America may learn something important from this experiment.

Godspeed, Croatia.

10 June 2007

Ethics and Medical Economics: Rationing Care

THERE ARE THREE ASPECTS OF MEDICAL ECONOMICS that concern me. The first is the "big picture" of macroeconomics and public policy. The second is the difficult and sometimes contentious interface between public policy and the patient with cancer. This essay focuses on the third of the trilogy by raising fundamental ethical questions: On what basis do we decide how to apply limited resources in a just manner? Who gets to decide?

I refer you to the *Journal of Clinical Oncology* special issue entitled, "Perspectives on the Cost of Cancer Care," for a broad review of the subject.[1] I especially recommend the article by Daniel Sulmasy[2] who addresses moral and ethical issues in medical cost containment.

First, do Americans pay too much for health care? A majority of economists would answer "yes." They believe our medical costs, 16% of the Gross Domestic Product (GDP), make us economically less competitive. Others disagree. The Stanford economist Victor Fuchs says we should not set an arbitrary GDP as enough spent on health care.[3] He believes that we should base spending on value gained, however one measures that, and control the rate of growth rather than the absolute amount. Robert Fogel, economist and Nobel Laureate at the University of Chicago, believes health care will continue to grow as a percent of GDP, reaching 25% by 2030.[4] He says that is perfectly OK, that an aging population and technological advances in health care will drive the economy like railroads did in the early 20th century. Nonetheless, there is a strong belief among many in economics, industry, and policy circles that medical costs should be contained. If that is the case, how should it be done?

"Cost Containment in Oncology Is a Moral Issue"

This is the first line in the article by Sulmasy[2]; I agree with it, though some economists and physicians do not. First, two terms: allocation is apportionment of ample or abundant resources; a pie is cut into the number of pieces needed for the guests at dinner. Rationing is a form of apportionment: limiting the individual portion of a scarce resource for the common good; gasoline is rationed during wartime to serve military needs. In a medical context, rationing is withholding a medical intervention that is of value to the patient for the good of others in the economic community. If one accepts that spending on health care must be contained and that the only practical way of doing so is restricting (rationing) the use of desired services (desired does not necessarily mean justified), then we are faced with the key question. Who decides? Even if one argues that health care resources are ample, but poorly distributed, the question of who decides remains.

Shall the Doctor, the Market, or the Government Decide?
Many believe that the doctor should decide because the individual circumstances are so varied and the decisions can be tailored to the specific situation. Proponents appeal to the practitioners' sense of the common good as a motive for bedside rationing, arguing that physicians must balance the needs of the patient with the needs of society and should take on this responsibility as part of their civic and medical duties. Many of us physicians are uncomfortable with that because the inherent conflict of interest compromises our duty, first and foremost, to the patient. Managed care organizations, believing that physicians were unlikely to ration resources for a common good, devised incentives – capitation, economic profiling, and bureaucratic barriers such as formulary restrictions and retrospective denials.

Others have strongly criticized bedside rationing as morally unjustified. Justice means all similar patients are offered a similar level of care. But patients in similar situations are likely to be treated differently by different physicians. Oncologists may or may not prescribe a very expensive new agent for identical patients with colon cancer, depending on whether they believe the extra month or two of life is worth the exorbitant cost. Also, in our health system, how would any individual oncologist know where the "savings" of withholding therapy would end up? It might simply result in greater corporate profit.

Offering financial incentives to doctors to contain costs also has its ethical problems. The patient thinks the doctor is making the decision in her best interests, when in fact he is simply the agent of the payer manipulating him to carry out the payers' wishes. This also forces the physician into a moral dilemma and may undermine her professionalism and create an air of distrust between doctor and patient.

A pure market approach would be untenable: If you don't have the money for chemotherapy, mortgage your house. If you can't afford vaccinations for your kids, borrow the money or go without. But today's health care insurance systems often use more nuanced market approaches, such as restricted formularies, co-pays, and deductibles. These practices are widely accepted today and may contain the cost of care to some extent. Or they may not contain overall costs, just the cost to the insurer or employer, and institutionalize the distribution of health care based on the patients' ability to pay. Both raise concerns for a just and moral process.

The government already decides to a large extent. In addition to the 35 million elderly Americans on Medicare in 2005, at least 38% of the non-elderly insured population (~100 million people) received publicly funded insurance. That includes those on Medicare and Medicaid, in the military, veterans, and other public sector employees. The total 135 million is nearly half of the United States population.[5] Gross also points out that the government is subsidizing health care in other ways. Employer-provided insurance premiums are exempt from federal and some state and local taxes. That amounts to about $208 billion or 35% of the cost of the premiums. This compares to $378 billion for Medicare and $180 billion for Medicaid in fiscal 2006. In the same article, Thomas Selden from the Agency for Healthcare Research and Quality is cited as estimating that in pure dollar terms public expenditures on health care made up 45% of all health care spending in 2004. In effect, nearly half of the population is covered by a single-payer government system.

From a moral viewpoint, government-funded health care has been administered with some success, but it too raises some ethical concerns. Government policies are subject to the whims of political dogmatism and the influence of interest-group lobbyists. It is also slow to change in response to medical advances and scientific evidence. The bureaucracy of government, however, is in some ways no worse than private insurance. The administrative cost of health care overall in the United States is 31% vs. 17% in Canada's national health system.

Decide by Cost-Effectiveness Analysis?
That leads us to cost-benefit or cost-effectiveness analyses (CEA). This science compares monetary cost to various outcomes such as years of life, quality of life, efficiency, and the like. Although he concedes that using CEA for decision analysis can be useful for informing complex decisions, Sulmasy believes there are bothersome problems of justice in actions derived from such studies, mainly because they are based on average outcomes that ignore the distribution.[2] His example is that CEA might recommend withholding a very expensive drug from a patient whose life would be extended 120 days in order to use the money for extending the life of 150 patients one day each. This approach also does not take into account such variables as different pain thresholds and patient preferences.

More important is whether a dollar cost can be used to value life. Sulmasy quotes Thomas Hobbes who believed that, "The value or worth of a man is, as with all other things, his price."[2] In contrast, Immanuel Kant believed that man "...has not merely a relative worth, i.e. a price, but an intrinsic worth, i.e. dignity." So Hobbes believed that a man's life was a commodity, perhaps very valuable, but still a commodity. Kant believed that man's value is intrinsic dignity, which is priceless.

However, Sulmasy points out that it is just as wrong to say life is priceless and that one should never limit any treatments for any reasons.[2] This view holds that any cancer treatment that has any chance of being effective no matter how small or costly must be given to patients and underwritten by third-party payers. He cites an article that reports a recent survey in which 78% of oncologists held this view. He believes this is largely due to "the wholesale abandonment of common sense reasoning in medicine." He points out that it once was common to say that the result of a study was "statistically significant but clinically unimportant. Such a common sense judgment is rarely heard today. Thus nearly every statistically significant improvement, no matter how small, is hailed as a breakthrough." We see this at every national meeting.

Decide by Common Sense?

Sulmasy is an advocate of a common sense approach, which basically involves withholding expensive treatments when there is no clinically significant advantage and not withholding an expensive treatment when studies show the advantage to be statistically significant and common sense indicates it is also clinically significant.[2] He goes into some detail about how to go about this. For each rationing decision concerning an expensive new treatment, he advocates an open, public, participatory process to set the limits. He admits this would not be easy, but believes that it offers the best chance for a just and fair result.

My own view is that Sulmasy's "common sense approach" is used at least occasionally today by many oncologists, though what is common sense to one may not be to another. I agree with him that oncology studies can and often do show that new agents provide a statistically significant advantage, but in practical terms offer very little. However, I am skeptical that any group could be formed to make that judgment and have a major influence on the practice of oncology. The Oregon Health Plan was similar to the proposed system and it failed.

In academia and in private practice, the psychology of both doctor and patient, our engrained American culture of individualism, and economic factors will continue to be the strongest influences on the cost of care. Unless industry, government and a substantial segment of the public agree that cost containment and a more just distribution of medical care is critical for the economic health and the common good of the country, cost containment will continue to be optional and arbitrary. Inability to pay and restricted access will be the tools for controlling medical costs, blunt tools that ignore justice.

25 March 2007

References

[1] Meropol NJ, Schulman KA, guest editors. Review issue "Perspective on the Cost of Cancer Care." *J Clin Oncol* 25:169-237, 2007

[2] Sulmasy DP. Cancer care, money, and the value of life: Whose justice? Which rationality? *J Clin Oncol* 25:217-222, 2007

[3] Fuchs VR: Health care expenditures reexamined. *Ann Int Med* 143: 76-78, 2005

[4] Kolata G: Making health care the engine that drives the economy. *The New York Times*, August 22, 2006

[5] Gross D: National health care? We're halfway there. *The New York Times*, December 3, 2006

Chapter 2
QUALITY OF CANCER CARE

There is no accepted national standard for assessing the quality of one's care. There is no reliable method for the patient to determine in advance who practices a better quality of care. Interest in this issue has grown in the past several years. This topic is dear to my heart. I have participated in several panels and written about the quality of care, including about the action that has been or should be taken.

QUALITY OF CANCER CARE

The Quality Waves Are Coming

AS LONG AS I CAN REMEMBER there has been talk about the quality of medical care. Over the past decade or two, hospitals have passed through an alphabet soup of "quality improvement" programs with remarkably little data to demonstrate sustained improvement of processes or outcomes. Community and academic ambulatory practices have been essentially absent from even that feeble process. A variety of factors have caused this state of affairs, including confusion over the definition of quality, the cost of sustaining programs, overweening confidence in the quality of one's practice, and fear of public comparison. But possibly the most important factor of all is the absence of any tangible consequences for participating or not.

But now the convergence of several strong forces is beginning to elevate the role of quality in medical care like a storm building in the Pacific that in time causes huge waves on distant shores, and sometimes causes tsunamis that wash away the unprepared. These forces include the following:

Release of influential studies by the Institute of Medicine[1]: "Ensuring Quality Cancer Care" (1999), "Enhancing Data Systems for Improving the Quality of Cancer Care" (2000), and "Crossing the Quality Chasm" (2001) all point out the major shortcomings in the quality of care in general, and the first two of cancer care in particular. These reports have prompted many substantive responses, including legislation in Congress and efforts to address the quality issue by the American Society of Clinical Oncology (ASCO) (see following).

Employers and payers, alarmed at the double-digit increases in the cost of care, but reluctant to deny access to necessary treatment, are focusing more and more on quality as a determinant of eligibility. Importantly, they define quality to include "value," i.e., cost and need, as well as medical excellence. The Leapfrog Group, a collaboration of medical directors of many Fortune 500 companies, presses quality issues more and more for their employees. Their principles include public disclosure of performance measures.

Dr. Robert Galvin, Director of Corporate Health Care at General Electric and a member of the Leapfrog Group, said at a recent summit meeting of the National

Comprehensive Cancer Network that it wouldn't be too long before "cost and quality data will become public." UnitedHealth Group, the country's largest health plan, pays for bone marrow transplantation for its members only at centers of excellence that, in their view, provide both medical excellence and value; they are planning a similar program for oncology in general. And the biggest payer of all, Centers for Medicare & Medicaid Services, already is applying quality measures to evaluate renal dialysis; it would be a short step to either steering patients to "quality" practices or "paying for quality," or both. Can oncology be far behind?

ASCO commissioned the Harvard School of Public Health and the Rand Corporation to assess the quality of cancer care in five metropolitan regions of the country. This study, the National Initiative in Cancer Care Quality (NICCQ), is well underway.[2]

ASCO also supports a pilot project for engaging practicing oncologists in a quality improvement program that is designed and monitored by the participating practitioners. The seven founding practices, called the Alpha Group, have almost completed testing the first set of questions by review of unselected charts and submitting the de-identified data online. The results were given back to each practice showing its performance relative to the unidentified remainder of the participants. Once testing of the process is complete, ASCO plans to invite all willing volunteers to participate further in the program.

Finally, cancer advocacy groups have always been interested in the quality of care. They have been represented in expert quality panels, such as those at the Institute of Medicine, and have informed and educated their constituents concerning various aspects of quality care. They have become an increasingly important and potent voice for high quality care.

So what is an oncologist to do when he or she learns that the "perfect storm" of the quality movement is gaining speed out there? My advice? The quality movement will impact your practice—community or academic, like it or not. If oncologists don't take leadership and participate in this arena, someone else will make decisions on what quality cancer care is and, perhaps, what third-party payers will pay for. In short, if we don't participate in credible, data-driven systems for self-examination that promote excellence in cancer care, we may be washed away by the big waves instead of riding them. But most of all, we should do it because the formal, systematic promotion of excellence in care in our practices is the right thing to do.

10 December 2003

References

[1] Institute of Medicine reports cited in this essay are available at www.nationalacademies.org/publications/

[2] Malin JL, Schneider EC, Epstein AM, et al: Results of the National Initiative for Cancer Care Quality: How can we improve the quality of cancer care in the United States? *J Clin Oncol* 24:626-634, 2006

The Quality Waves Are Coming – What to Do?

IN THE PREVIOUS ESSAY (*see pp 54-55*), I described how a convergence of factors is building the quality movement into a "perfect storm." Several reports from the Institute of Medicine are critical of the quality of cancer care; Congress is considering legislation on the quality of cancer care; payers and employers are increasingly insisting on value (cost and need) as well as medical excellence; the American Society of Clinical Oncology (ASCO) has mounted two programs to assess and improve cancer care; and advocates for quality cancer care grow in influence. These forces are primed to make big waves across oncology.

I said I believed that this movement would have a profound impact on oncologists and on the operation and economics of their practices. I urged oncologists to take a leadership role in the quality arena because if they didn't, someone else would. But more important, because an evidence-based, systematic process of self-examination that promotes excellent cancer care was the right thing to do.

Before providing examples of how one might proceed to develop a quality program in practice, let's dispense with several issues that might bog down the effort.

First, I am not suggesting yet another formal academic study of quality; there are more than enough practice guidelines, documented standards of care, and widely accepted "common sense" standards available for use. Rather, I suggest a modest, but practical and systematic, program suitable for community and academic oncologists.

Second, I will not argue over the definitions of quality or how many qualities will fit on the head of a pin. One may choose from a wide variety of standards. My own benchmarks of quality care are simple:
- Care I would want my family to have
- Care given with skill, sensitivity, efficiency, and economy
- Care based on peer-reviewed data or *validated* experience
- Care given in a serious learning environment that includes clinical trials
- Care recorded fully and accurately

And third, many oncologists view guidelines as an infringement on their judgment, so let's deal directly with specific objections to starting a quality initiative, followed by my rejoinder to each.

- "I already give quality care." *Show me the data!*
- "I am too busy. *Would you say that if the patient were your mother or son?*"
- "It will cost money, staff time, and more paperwork." *Yes it will, more in the short run.*
- "I have no say in what quality is or what measures will be used." *You can learn and choose your own, or join an ongoing program.*
- "I fear the inappropriate use of the data by the public, competitors or the government, with the possible loss of income." *Join colleagues in a quality program that controls its own data.*

So how does one start? It is useful to think of quality measures as falling into one of three classes: structure, process, or outcomes. An example of structure might be to include the pathology report or a chemotherapy flow sheet in the patient's chart. Process might be to ask every patient in relapse and record at each visit whether he/she has pain. Outcome could be length of remission, toxicity, or patient satisfaction.

Depending on the size and site of the practice, chart rounds and tumor boards can help control quality, but objective, data-driven measures are essential to enable the tracking of progress, or lack of it. One might select guidelines like those published by ASCO concerning the use of erythropoietin or other growth factors and regularly review a number of unselected charts to see whether one's practice complies, and if not, why not. One could do the same with the National Comprehensive Cancer Network guidelines for chemotherapy, pain control, or the sequencing of therapy. Whatever one chooses, it must be done systematically, perhaps with new measures every 4 to 6 months and the repetition of older measures annually.

For some, it may be easiest to join an ongoing program at a hospital or neighboring practice. ASCO's practitioner-driven quality program is open to any willing volunteers. In addition to being led by actively practicing oncologists under the aegis of the Health Services Committee, the program has several virtues that may make it an attractive option. The quality measures are devised and tested by a group of seven practices of different sizes and from all parts of the country, known as the Alpha Group. The user-friendly data collection system set up by the ASCO Information Technology Department uses a slick electronic data entry system to collect and collate the de-identified data. This allows one to compare one's practice to many other unidentified practices from around the country. (In the spirit of full disclosure, I participate in the development of this program.)

Other professional organizations such as the American College of Surgeons and the American Society of Therapeutic Radiology and Oncology also have quality improvement programs. Information is available on their websites.

The precise form of a quality program is less important than the result one hopes to achieve: that oncologists take leadership, embrace guidelines, and use quality and outcome measures to create a culture of self-examination to promote excellence in care; in short, to create a practice environment that we would want for our family and ourselves if one of us were the patient.

25 December 2003

Assessing the Quality of Cancer Care at the State Level

THE QUALITY OF EFFORTS TO CONTROL CANCER and manage the patient with cancer continues to be a growing concern by many, including me. In prior essays I have described a series of reports issued by the National Cancer Policy Board (NCPB) of the Institute of Medicine (IOM) on the quality of cancer care, efforts by the American Society of Clinical Oncology to examine and promote excellence in care, the growing interest of insurers in "pay for performance" that includes quality measures, and a variety of institutional activities in this arena. And now the State of Georgia has begun an important effort to address the quality of cancer care at the state level.

In 2001 with funds promised from the tobacco settlement, the State of Georgia formed the Georgia Cancer Coalition (GCC; www.georgiacancer.org) with the expressed purpose of reducing the burden of cancer for citizens of the state. The GCC has started a variety of programs that support research, education, cancer centers, and community activities. In 2003 the leadership of the GCC expressed interest in finding a way to gauge Georgia's progress in improving the quality of its cancer services and in reducing cancer-related morbidity and mortality. With financial support from the Woodruff Foundation, the GCC commissioned the IOM to develop a framework for measuring progress statewide.

The charge from the GCC was that a measure set should be pertinent to the mission and goals of the GCC, in a form that is reasonable to implement, and drawn from established clinical guidelines or quality measures already in use. The GCC's mission includes addressing issues across the complete scope of cancer care and services, from prevention, diagnosis, and treatment through palliative care and survivorship.

In the fall of 2003 the IOM formed the Committee on Assessing Improvements in Cancer Care in Georgia. It consisted of 11 individuals with expertise in various aspects of cancer research and care, epidemiology, health services research, health care policy, state cancer databases, nursing, and quality improvement research and implementation. (Full disclosure–I had the privilege of serving on this committee.) Virtually all of the research and writing was done by two members of the NCPB-IOM staff, Jill Eden and

Elizabeth Brown. The committee met in person only once, but communicated often via conference calls and e-mail. The committee consulted a large number of other experts in the state of Georgia and around the country, including representatives of the Centers for Disease Control, the National Cancer Institute, and the Rollins School of Public Health at Emory University.

The mission of the committee was to develop a set of quality-of-care measures that could be used by states—Georgia in particular, but more broadly applicable, as well—to assess progress in improving cancer-related services and in reducing cancer morbidity and mortality; to address economic, geographic, racial, and ethnic disparities in cancer care; to inform the governor, state legislature, and executive branch of GCC's progress; to contribute to quality improvement initiatives and health education; and to educate the state's health care community and the general public about cancer. The measures had to be validated in some way and the data largely obtainable from existing data sources. Measures fell into one of five categories: prevention; early detection; diagnostics; treatment (including pain control and end-of-life care); and cross-cutting measures such as patient satisfaction and racial disparities. This structure allows GCC, based on its experience over time, to drop, change, replace, or add measures while maintaining the categorical spectrum.

Throughout the process the committee evaluated several characteristics of candidate measures, mainly importance, supporting evidence and feasibility of collection. It was decided that at this time measures that were tumor-specific would be limited to the "big four," lung, breast, colorectal, and prostate cancer. Cross-cutting measures, such as patient satisfaction and racial disparities, would apply to any form of cancer.

The report was completed in late 2004 and was then sent by the IOM to seven expert reviewers and two referees. They offered many helpful suggestions for clarification which were incorporated into the final version of the report. The report officially passed final review in February 2005. Final copies are available from National Academies Press and the report is readable online at www.nap.edu.[1]

The following is a brief listing of the 52 quality measures.

Prevention Measures: adult smoking rate; adolescent smoking rate; number of smokers advised to quit; smokers who are recommended pharmacotherapy to assist in quitting; adult obesity rate; cancer incidence (all sites and specifically breast, lung, colorectal, and prostate).

Early Detection: breast cancer screening rate; colorectal cancer screening rate; proportion of breast cancer cases diagnosed at an early stage; incidence of advanced-stage breast cancer; incidence of advanced-stage colorectal cancer.

Diagnosing Cancer: timely breast cancer biopsy; use of needle biopsy before breast cancer surgery; tumor-free surgical margins in breast-conserving surgery; appropriate histological assessment of Stages I and II breast cancer and colorectal cancer; pathology laboratories that report College of American Pathologists data elements on cancer specimens in general and on breast, colorectal, lung, and prostate cancers in particular; breast, lung, colorectal, and prostate cancer cases in which cancer stage was established and recorded before chemotherapy and radiation.

Treating Cancer: patients with cancer who participate in clinical trials; frequency of inappropriate hormone therapy before radical prostatectomy for prostate cancer; appropriate doses of external-beam radiation therapy for prostate cancer; appropriate hormonal therapy with external-beam radiation therapy for high-risk prostate cancer; adjuvant radiation after breast-conserving surgery for women under age 70 with invasive breast cancer; adjuvant hormonal therapy for hormone-receptor positive invasive breast cancer; adjuvant combination chemotherapy for women under age 71 with hormone-receptor-negative Stage I to III breast cancer; adjuvant chemotherapy after surgery for Stage III colon cancer; follow-up mammography after treatment for Stage 0-III breast cancer; follow-up colonoscopy after treatment for Stage I-III colorectal cancer.

This category also includes: patients with cancer who are regularly assessed for pain; prevalence of more than minor pain among patients with cancer; cancer deaths in hospice per 100 cancer deaths; cancer patients who receive hospice care for at least 7 days; 5- and 10-year relative survival rates for female breast, colorectal, lung, and prostate cancers; cancer deaths per 100,000 persons per year for breast, colorectal, lung, and prostate cancers and for all cancers.

The report also recommends that Georgia invest in developing surveys to capture information on the experience of patients with cancer, e.g., functional status, treatment-related symptoms, satisfaction, access, out-of-pocket costs, barriers to services, and timeliness of services. The GCC should also improve existing data systems to evaluate disparities in cancer care and services by standardizing race and ethnicity data enabling the comparison of all the above measures by such categories.

When fully implemented and in place for a period of time, these measures will enable the GCC to track progress, or the lack of it, in controlling cancer and its effects. Implementation will not be easy or cheap, but it will be feasible and, in my view, will provide data for wide-ranging analysis and research, and also identify opportunities for intervention and improvement. The leadership of the State of Georgia is to be commended for conceiving and funding this project, a project that is unique and likely to be copied in some form by other states.

10 April 2005

Reference
[1] Eden J, Simone JV (eds): Assessing the quality of cancer care: An approach to measurement in Georgia. Washington, DC, The National Academies Press, 2005. (www.nationalacademies.org/publications/)

Policy Efforts to Improve the Quality of Cancer Care

IT IS A GREAT BLESSING IN LIFE to be, by chance or design, part of a group of people that makes one better: more loving, selfless, or generous; more open-minded, insightful, or productive. One of the many such blessings I have enjoyed has been membership on the National Cancer Policy Board (NCPB) of the Institute of Medicine (IOM), which was instrumental in raising my interest and that of many others in taking steps to improve the general quality of cancer care.

At the suggestion of Dr. Richard Klausner, director of the National Cancer Institute (NCI) at the time, the Board was founded in 1997 to issue independent policy reports on important topics in cancer care and research. The NCI had been asked to do such work, but Dr. Klausner believed it was ill-suited to the task, being a research organization and part of federal government. The NCI committed the bulk of the funds—unrestricted, no strings attached—to support the work.

The reports of the Board (and all the committees of the IOM) are intended to provide an independent, objective review of important issues and, in some reports, to recommend a series of policy actions. Reports are rigorously peer-reviewed by experts and refined before release. The target audiences are federal and local governments and their various agencies, academicians, the health and research industries, and the public.

I have benefited enormously from my 8 years on the Board. I have met and learned from a lot of accomplished, smart, and interesting Board members, as well as from those invitees who provided formal and informal analyses. That broad expertise has exposed me to views and insights I might not otherwise have experienced. The ever-renewing membership has included basic, clinical and population researchers, lawyers, economists, leaders in the health care and bio-pharma industries, nurses, ethicists, chief executive officers of research, charitable and commercial organizations, and representatives of patient advocacy groups. The striking diversity has been a wonderful asset to the Board's productivity and insight. And the IOM staffers have been a pleasure to know and work with; they did most of the writing and other heavy lifting for our activities and, in many ways small and large, they made us look good

But most important, the reports of the Board have been well received and useful, and several have had a major impact on the policies of organizations, both private and public. All the reports, workshops, and background papers can be found at www.iom.edu/ncpb or through Google by simply entering "National Cancer Policy Board." The Board's website appears in the top ten of all search engines when using the terms "cancer" plus "policy," and is first at Google. A summary of some of the reports of the Board follows.

During its first 3 years, the Board issued three full reports:
- *Ensuring Quality Cancer Care* (1999)—more on this below
- *Taking Action to Reduce Tobacco Use* (1998)
- *State Programs Can Reduce Tobacco Use* (2000)

Also during the first 3 years, two IOM committee studies were initiated under the aegis of the Board resulting in reports on:
- Extending Medicare Reimbursement in Clinical Trials. This was released 12/15/99 and led to the President's Executive Memorandum and the Health Care Financing Administration's National Coverage Decision establishing a national policy for Medicare and Medicare+Choice payment for care associated with trials.
- Mammography and Beyond: *Developing Technologies for the Early Detection of Breast Cancer*. This report reviewed current technologies under exploration or development for detecting breast cancer and was released with a companion lay version 3/8/01 and subsequently underwent extensive dissemination nationwide.

Ensuring Quality Cancer Care also led to the establishment by the Department of Health and Human Services the Quality of Cancer Care Committee (QC3) and stimulated quality of care projects by the American Society of Clinical Oncology. It generated other quality efforts by the Board, as noted below. It was also widely distributed to Congress, the Executive Branch, academia, all the partners of the National Dialogue on Cancer (where it formed the basis of Dialogue recommendations), and the public where it was frequently referenced and proved influential. A number of new initiatives were undertaken by the NCI as a result of this report, including efforts with the Agency for Healthcare Research and Quality and the National Quality Forum to develop core indicators of quality of cancer care.

Much of the Board's subsequent work built on *Ensuring Quality Cancer Care*. The Board began by focusing on four projects expanding on the major emphasis of that report. These have been released as follows:
- *Enhancing Data Systems to Improve the Quality of Cancer Care* (released 10/4/00).
- *Interpreting the Volume-Outcome Relationship in the Context of Health Care Quality: A Workshop Summary* (released 12/6/00).

- *Interpreting the Volume-Outcome Relationship in the Context of Cancer Care: A White Paper* (released 7/12/01).
- *Improving Palliative Care for Cancer* (released 6/19/01) which included English and Spanish short lay versions.

The Board has completed a number of workshops and reports that represent additional offspring of *Ensuring Quality Cancer Care* and its sequels including:
- *Fulfilling the Potential of Cancer Prevention and Early Detection*. This was a major report with significant input from the NCI, Centers for Disease Control, and the academic prevention and screening communities (released 3/10/03).
- *Describing Death in America: What We Need to Know*. This followed the original report on palliative care that examined data systems on end-of-life patients in a study commissioned from RAND and a workshop held 10/10/01 (released 4/3/03).
- *Cancer Survivorship: Improving Care and Quality of Life*. This was a major project with broad input from the NCI, survivorship, and academic communities. It was divided into cancer survivorship reports in children (released 8/26/03) and adults (in preparation, 2004). An additional survivorship report (released 1/28/04) was based on a workshop held 10/28-29/02, *Meeting Psychosocial Needs of Women with Breast Cancer*.

The Board's attention also focused on cancer research:
- A series of background papers and a short report grew out of a project originally titled *Shortening the Timeline for New Cancer Treatments*. They include: *Making Better Drugs for Children with Cancer; Human Tissue Samples and Cancer Drug Development: Barriers and Opportunities;* and *Technology Transfer Among Government, Universities, and Industry: Building More Effective Relationships*. The final paper, *Federal Agency Roles in Cancer Drug Development from Preclinical Research to New Drug Approval: The National Cancer Institute and Food and Drug Administration* (in review, 2005), examines ways to improve the efficiency and timeliness of cancer drug development.
- *Large-Scale Biomedical Science: Exploring Strategies for Future Research*. This is an exploration of issues for research done as large, costly, capital intense, multi-site, collaborative projects with a focus on cancer research which was released 6/19/03 and distributed at the National Institutes of Health Biomedical Engineering Consortium (Catalyzing Team Science) meeting, 6/24/03.

The Board took a leadership role in the relationship of the IOM with the Georgia Cancer Coalition (GCC), a multi-year effort of the State of Georgia (tobacco settlement funds) to improve cancer care, research, and education in that state. In 2005 the NCPB released a report commissioned by the GCC, *Assessing the Quality of Cancer Care – an Approach to Measurement in Georgia*. In addition to helping Georgia evaluate its statewide cancer improvement programs, the report serves as a model for other states to use in evaluating their own cancer programs.

In 2005, the Board released *Improving Mammography Quality Standards*, a report that recommends improvements for the reauthorization of the federal Mammography Quality Standards Act, which was requested by the Congress, and *Cancer Control in Low- and Middle-Income Countries*, which proposes ways in which such countries can mount cancer control programs most suited to their particular circumstances.

So why am I recalling my experience with the NCPB at this time? In a sense, this is a nostalgic eulogy. The Board ceased to exist in 2005 due to a lack of funds. My sadness is tempered by the remarkable record of its accomplishment; its reports will live on to inform and inspire others. It is also tempered by the formation of a cancer forum, which unlike the NCPB will include representatives of government agencies and will not issue reports, but will retain a cancer-specific focus at the IOM.

Membership on the Board was an eye-opening and fulfilling experience and I am proud of all the members, staff, and reports. But especially, I am proud of its impact on raising awareness and stimulating action toward improving the quality of cancer care.

10 February 2005

The Many Faces of Quality Cancer Care

I HAVE PREVIOUSLY OFFERED MY VIEWS of why quality of cancer care has not yet become a major priority on the agendas of caregivers, health care organizations, payers, and government. My experience at three quality symposia in the last 2 weeks has given me additional perspectives on the complexity of the issue. The three audiences and sites of the symposia were: a local organization of oncologists in New York; an array of professionals and staffers participating in a state-wide cancer control effort in Seattle; and in Boston, an eclectic medical group of academics, payers, and others focused on improving quality by changing the care system.

At the first meeting I spoke to an association of oncologists about the forces moving us to improving the quality of cancer care with accountability. I then described the Quality Oncology Practice Initiative (QOPI) as an example of a voluntary, practice-based effort for comparing one's performance to many others.[1] Although some in the audience expressed support of the idea, several very vocal medical oncologists attacked the whole concept. I had been accustomed to some disagreements with the QOPI approach based on its perceived value or effectiveness, but this was quite different.

I will quote (approximately) some of the comments: "This is a waste of time; you need to do something about reimbursement." "In my office if I told my nurse to collect this information, she would say she has no time." "All you are doing is giving the insurance companies more ammunition to harass us. I've been in practice 30 years and I don't need any guidelines or quality measures and some stupid high school dropout at the insurance company telling me I can't give this or that treatment." This went on for 15 minutes despite my protestations that the QOPI information is controlled by participating physicians, and that I really couldn't do anything about their reimbursement woes.

I learned afterward that the vocal vehemence came from older practitioners who are in one- or two-person practices in typical telephone-booth-sized offices in Manhattan. I was told by my host that these small practices of docs in their 60s and 70s are suffering more from the constriction of reimbursement and the sea changes in health care, partly due to the economics of small practices and partly due simply to resistance to any change. Thus, quality improvement is not high on their lists of priorities.

My second experience that week was in Seattle at a gathering of about 150 professionals and staffers working to develop a state-wide quality assessment-improvement program. There were several speakers, including representatives of the National Comprehensive Cancer Network, the National Quality Forum, Texas Oncology PA, the National Cancer Database and cancer registrars. I gave a talk about QOPI as well as a talk about the report of the Institute of Medicine, "Assessing the Quality of Cancer Care: An Approach to Measurement in Georgia," which I had co-edited. The audience was engaged, asked many questions for clarification or rose to support or challenge some of the positions taken by the speakers. All the questions and comments were aimed at understanding how they could best use their talents and resources to develop their program for assessing the quality of cancer care in the State of Washington. They had attended the meeting with that goal in mind.

My third experience a few days later was in Boston. Dr. Laura Esserman, a professor of surgery and an expert in breast cancer at the University of California San Francisco (UCSF), organized the workshop, "Advancing the Agenda for Quality in Medicine." The aim was to share ideas that would lead to a new model of cancer care delivery that could be implemented and tested initially for patients with breast cancer at UCSF.

The speakers were leaders in academic medicine, health services research, organizational research, Medicare, voluntary organizations, advocacy groups, large employers, health plans, and foundations. The talks were fascinating, some revealing areas under study to a degree that I have not been aware of, such as new ways of supporting patient choice by developing profiles of values and general preferences before the choices need to be made. The talks included those that addressed the latest demonstration project in cancer of the Center of Medicare and Medicaid Services, innovative databases for cancer care, the redesign of the process of diagnosis and evaluation, a panel discussion by very articulate cancer survivors, who were also health care or business professionals, about their assessments of the system of care they received, and others.

The tone of the meeting was one of inquiry and innovation, searching for key factors for developing better models of care. I gave a talk that described lessons to be learned from the system of care in pediatric oncology and why the latter has been more successful, and I also talked again about QOPI. The outcome was the identification and discussion of important issues when developing new care models. Also, there was a movement in my own breakout group to find a way to get Centers for Medicare & Medicaid Services, employers, and payers to require the reporting of cancer staging, particularly before the initial treatment.

The fact that these three meetings occurred over less than 2 weeks caused me to think about the variety of landscapes and viewpoints of quality that must be recognized if one is to be successful at "Advancing the Agenda." There must be many additional "faces" of quality that I have not experienced.

Aside from observing and learning about the differing viewpoints of quality, both theoretical and practical, this concentrated experience made the following impressions on me. First, there are many more talented people working on novel aspects of quality care than I had realized. This was most encouraging. Second, because of the complexity of quality medical care, this distributed focus on many different aspects and models is a good thing and should be encouraged and supported by granting agencies, payers, and providers. There will not be a single solution to achieving a sustained and imbedded effort in quality improvement, even in a relatively circumscribed area like oncology. Many approaches will fail but, with perseverance, successful ones are sure to emerge.

Finally, the experience convinced me once again that the key to the systematic improvement of the quality of care is the leadership and innovation of physicians. Certainly, enlightened payers, health plans, and hospitals are necessary, but the role of the physician remains central to the process. We are the ombudsmen for our patients and we known them best; that puts the responsibility squarely on our shoulders.

25 February 2006

Reference

[1] McNiff K: The Quality Oncology Practice Initiative: Assessing and improving care within the medical oncology practice. *J Oncol Prac* 2:26-30, 2006 (*see also www.asco.org*)

Pay for Performance

"PAY FOR PERFORMANCE" (P4P) IS A HOT TOPIC in medicine today. It is a response to the increasing cost of medical care, medical errors, the wide geographic variation in cost, and evidence of overuse and underuse of medical products and services. These issues are not new, but they are now fueled by the growing quality of care movement. This alignment of social forces potentially provides a rare opportunity to improve the quality of care and offers payers an ethical basis for controlling costs, since many believe that high quality care is less expensive in the long run. So, exactly what is P4P and what implications might it have for the future practice of medicine?

P4P is the payment of a reimbursement premium for meeting certain measurable practice goals. This has been implemented mainly in primary care practices. Clinical measures include high compliance with the desired frequency of immunizations, Pap smears, mammographic and colonoscopy screening, and the use of hemoglobin A1c for screening and management of diabetes. "Patient experience" measures often include the timeliness of care, doctor-patient communication, and the coordination of care. Some models also include information technology measures, such as using electronic medical records or electronic aids for more efficient diagnosis and management. Areas assessed can be weighted, e.g., 50% for clinical, 30% for patient experience, and 20% for information technology, with an added bonus for aggregate compliance and a formal feedback mechanism for improvement.

Much of the above can be found in greater detail at the website of a California not-for-profit organization, Integrated Health care Association (IHA) www.iha.org, which is highly recommended. The IHA model and how it came to be is particularly instructive.

The California HealthCare Foundation (CHCF) website, www.chcf.org, provides the following background. "The Pay for Performance initiative is a statewide program that focuses on developing and evaluating financial and non-financial incentives to improve the quality of health care being delivered in California. The CHCF has provided support, within the context of the national Robert Wood Johnson Foundation's "Rewarding Results" program, to the Integrated Healthcare Association (IHA) to lead one of the most comprehensive and ambitious programs in the country. IHA is composed of top decision-makers from the major health care stakeholder groups in California. Members include health plans, physician groups, hospital systems, researchers, businesses or purchasing groups, and consumers. CHCF is also supporting RAND and the University of California, Berkeley to evaluate the impact of the IHA Pay for Performance initiative in California.

"The Pay for Performance measurement set has been adopted wholly or substantially by six major health plans in California—Aetna, Blue Cross, Blue Shield, CIGNA, Health Net, and PacifiCare. In 2005, Western Health Advantage will also adopt the IHA performance measurement set. These plans have introduced the program for their commercial health maintenance organization members, which represent about 7 million enrollees in California. In 2003 more than 220 physician organizations participated in at least one of the three performance measurement domains—clinical performance, patient experience, and information technology.

"Pay for Performance data collection and aggregation is performed by the National Committee of Quality Assurance (NCQA). All six participating health plans have submitted clinical data to NCQA. A number of physician groups have chosen to augment this information with self-reported data. The health plans are using these data to make quality performance incentive payments to physician organizations. While calculations are still underway, in 2004 these payments are estimated to total approximately $50 million. Final numbers will be announced in July 2005."

Several features of this P4P program's development by IHA demonstrate insight and prudence. First, the initial funding and continued support comes from not-for-profit sources, i.e., foundations. Second, all the stakeholders were at the planning table from day 1—physicians, hospitals, health plans, patient representatives, businesses, and researchers—and the process was facilitated by individuals with no monetary or professional stake in the outcome. Third, a strong research and evaluation team was in place from the start of the project. This model has much to teach others who wish to develop P4P programs.

Center for Medicare & Medicaid Services (CMS) has a broad array of P4P initiatives in place or under development www.cms.hhs.gov. The furthest along is the Hospital Quality Initiative that uses 10 quality measures. CMS also has a series of demonstration projects for hospitals and physicians to address safety and variations in cost and care, and other projects focused on care guidelines, disease management, and evidence-based measures.

In addition, many professional societies and other health care organizations have spoken on P4P. The American Medical Association, the American College of Physicians, the American Academy of Family Practice, and the Joint Commission on Accreditation of Health Care Organizations have each published discussions, principles, or guidelines concerning the implementation of P4P.

But what about oncology? Until recently, there was relatively little movement in oncology and other subspecialty groups toward P4P, but that is changing. CMS is working with the American Society of Clinical Oncology (ASCO) on a P4P demonstration project. It is hard to predict the outcome of these nascent discussions, but a demonstration would likely be consistent with the other P4P activities of CMS.

ASCO's Quality Oncology Practice Initiative (QOPI), which is a voluntary, physician-run quality improvement program for oncology practitioners, is easily adaptable to a P4P program. Both CMS and private health plans are interested in working with QOPI for P4P initiatives. At his testimony on 27 July 2005 before the Congressional Ways and Means Committee chaired by Representative Nancy Johnson of Connecticut, Dr. Mark McClellan, (then) Director of CMS, specifically mentioned QOPI as a model that could be adapted by CMS for P4P.

QOPI now has 23 practices in the demonstration phase that have volunteered to review a set of recent charts twice a year. The results are graphed and returned to the practices so each may see how it is performing compared to colleagues elsewhere. The data are entered online, usually by data managers or nurses in the practices. The estimated cost to the practice for the time of the data manager is $400-$800 for each chart review, depending on the pay scale and the person's experience. At its August meeting, the Board of Directors of ASCO approved a budget for moving beyond the demonstration phase and open QOPI membership to the practice of any ASCO member. The plan is to notify all ASCO members of the opportunity to join QOPI. After completing the application, the first chart review for the expanded group was scheduled for March 2006. [Over 200 practices participated in the Spring 2007 data collection.]

A new approach to P4P is at an embryonic stage: P4P for profit. Entrepreneurs are planning to enlist practices in companies that provide the means to take advantage of the P4P system to profit from the reimbursement premium by dealing directly with insurance companies and also by selling the information on the evolving prescription patterns to pharmaceutical companies.

Finally, is P4P a good thing? The goals of improving both the quality of care and accountability are unassailable. But many questions remain. Will health plans become the arbiter of quality? Will the pot of money be the same so that the premium paid to one group is taken from another group that may not even be participating in P4P, having no chance to compete? As with any new project, there are apt to be mistakes and stumbles and any program of this complexity is likely to leave plenty of room for mischief by both payers and providers. But with all its uncertainty and warts, P4P seems to be a prudent and potentially revolutionary process for improving both the quality and financial discipline of health care. Even modest inroads in those two areas could have a major positive impact for patients and the country.

10 September 2005

QUALITY OF CANCER CARE

Pay for Performance – Dead or Alive?

A RECENT DECREASE IN THE CHATTER about P4P has led some to believe that the concept is dead or at least on life support. But two recent articles contest that belief; one describes a successful pilot project by Medicare with physician groups and the other describes a novel—and surprising—twist on the concept.

Reed Abelson in *The New York Times* reported preliminary results of a Medicare pilot study scheduled to run from 2005 to 2008 that involves ten medical practice groups.[1] They are described as "large, sophisticated organizations, with substantial experience in electronic health records or other systems known to improve patient care." (The last five words have precious little data to support them.) Medicare compared the hospital and doctor bills for the 224,000 patients treated by the ten practices with those of other doctors practicing in the same geographic areas to determine whether there were financial savings. Doctors also had to meet certain quality criteria for diseases such as diabetes.

Data from the first year of the project demonstrated that all ten practices showed improvement in cost savings and quality of care. However, only two groups improved enough to meet the threshold required to earn bonus cash payments. The University of Michigan Faculty Practice and the Marshfield Clinic in Wisconsin were paid a total bonus of $7.3 million for saving Medicare $8.5 million. Medicare has not yet calculated the savings of all ten practices, but the latter claim they saved Medicare $21 million in the first year.

Several of the practices have devised novel, money-saving processes as a result of the study, such as reducing unnecessary visits to specialists, reducing inpatient admissions, and follow-up by phone within 24 hours of patients discharged from the hospital or the emergency room to be sure they understood their medications and treatment plan.

Although Medicare officials were quoted as being enthusiastic about the project and predicted that all the participants would eventually receive bonus payments, some participants reported that the slow accumulation and reporting of data makes it difficult to respond to the potential financial advantages. This led at least one participant from the University of Michigan to doubt that the financial model is viable. There are also worries about the lack of reimbursement for services that save Medicare money, but cost the practices money that is not reimbursed.

Abelson also raises a critical issue that may confound such approaches: how to motivate individual physicians.[1] The experiment rewards organizations, not the individual doctor "who must actually insure that the patient gets a flu shot or goes to the right specialist." It is also not a simple thing to implement such a system in smaller, less corporate practices that do not have the resources to make some of the changes or for whom the potential bonus may be insufficient to motivate participation.

The second *New York Times* article, by Andrew Pollack, is entitled "Pricing Pills by the Results," and it is intriguing.[2] Johnson & Johnson has proposed that Britain's National Health Service pay for the cancer drug bortezomib (Velcade) for myeloma, *but only for people who benefit from the medicine*. GlaxoSmithKline has made similar arrangements with other European countries. Pollack sees this as a potential new version of pay-for-performance which is being called "risk-sharing." (This reminds me of reading that in ancient Chinese medicine, the doctor was paid only if the patient got better; what a concept!)

As the article points out, this would be very difficult to implement in the United States. Dr. Lee Newcomer of United HealthCare comments: "State regulations and marketplace pressures make it virtually impossible for an insurer to refuse to pay for a drug that has been approved by the FDA, regardless of its price."

Nonetheless, United HealthCare has entered a "risk-sharing" arrangement with Genomic Health, which sells a genetic test for patients with early breast cancer to determine if they would benefit from chemotherapy. United HealthCare has agreed to pay for the test for 18 months to see if it is of value. If too many women are still receiving chemotherapy even if the test suggests they don't need it, the insurer will negotiate for a lower price on the grounds that the test does not have the intended effect on practice. "The point is to try to make the manufacturer responsible for how their product is used in the medical marketplace," says Newcomer.[2]

Cigna Pharmacy Management is trying to persuade makers of cholesterol-lowering drugs to agree to pay for the medical expenses of patients who suffer heart attacks even though they have been steadfastly taking their medicine.

What are we to make of all this activity by insurers and pharmaceutical companies? Call me cynical, but I seriously doubt that they are taking these steps out of the goodness of their hearts. It is no secret why most of this activity is taking place in European nations with national health insurance. The central control gives those countries enormous bargaining power with pharmaceutical companies; Medicare is expressly forbidden by law to bargain over prices with pharmaceutical companies. Johnson & Johnson worked out the deal in Britain after the National Health Service declined to pay for Velcade until a deal was worked out to limit the number of doses based on the failure to respond adequately. Insurers are battling the increasing costs of care with innovative approaches. Some may even work. But throughout the article ran a thread of pessimism that any such innovations could succeed on a significant scale in this country.

So is P4P alive or dead? I would say it is very much alive, but it may be like the shmoo in Al Capp's old comic strip, Li'l Abner. These four-foot tall mozzarella-shaped beings were always getting in the way and they had a peculiar quality. Every time someone hit one to get it out of the way, it broke into many more little shmoos. P4P may be like that. P4P may get screwed up, especially in this country, and like the shmoos may just get in the way and not be very useful.

But I think it will live on though its ultimate shape and variations will probably surprise us as much as Li'l Abner.

25 August 2007

References
[1] Abelson R: Shift in health-cost is said to show promise. *The New York Times*, July 12, 2007
[2] Pollack A: Pricing pills by the results. *The New York Times*, July 14, 2007

Slow Pace of Improvement in the Quality of Medical Care

IN 1999 THE INSTITUTE OF MEDICINE (IOM) RELEASED the first of a series of reports, "Ensuring Quality Cancer Care," that described the shortcomings of cancer care in America and offered a list of recommendations for addressing them. At about the same time, the IOM also released two widely publicized reports, "To Err Is Human," which described the high frequency of medical errors in the United States, and "Crossing the Quality Chasm," which called for an overhaul of the health care delivery system because of its waste, inefficiency, and spotty quality.

Those reports have led to several studies of the quality of cancer care, including the Cancer Care and Outcomes Research and Surveillance (CanCORS) project by the National Cancer Institute and the National Initiative on Cancer Care Quality (NICCQ) sponsored by the American Society of Clinical Oncology (ASCO). They also have led to a proliferation of "quality" committees, alliances, and working groups. But one may now ask what progress has been made since those reports in improving the quality of health care, not just studying or talking about it.

Dr. Donald Berwick, President of the Institute for Healthcare Improvement, was interviewed by Dr. Robert Galvin, Director of Global Healthcare for General Electric, in 2005 about progress in improving health care quality (www.HealthAffairs.org).[1] Berwick has been an inspirational leader in the quality movement for many years and is an active member of the IOM and a participant in framing its reports. Here are excerpts from that interview.

"The pace and improvement of care itself are still very disappointing. Despite a lot of attention and push, and despite the presence of a few organizations that are starting to really change care, it has not become the mainstream agenda to change care properly yet. So we've still got a long way to go."

When asked whether the few organizations that are trying to change have the capacity to do so, he responded: "Do they have the physical and financial resources to make changes? We already have a bloated system with tremendous excess capacity. So we don't really have a resource issue here, in my mind, with a few exceptions... Can people in the workforce—doctors, nurses, receptionists, therapists—change their own work? Are they capable of making innovations happen? The answer is, No, they're not. We've never trained the workforce to change its work...And all the successful [organizations] are investing in retraining their own staffs."

"[Workforce capacity] is not a primary problem, though; it's a secondary problem. The capability that is key to the proper allocation of resources and development of the proper workforce is leadership, and that's where we still lack traction... There is a deficiency of will and ambition in the major centers of power in the delivery of health care in America. We do not have a shared aim to raise the bar in performance. That's the problem...you need insiders. And where would you go other than the board and senior executive suite?...Boards have tended to be seats of honor, not stewardship. Board members are volunteers so it's not their day job to be guiding the organization. They trust their doctors, and they're intimidated by the technology and the technical aspects of care. As a result, they do not inspect the core performance characteristics of the organization that they are stewards of, other than finance, and that's the problem."

The interview then turns from health care organizations and their leaders to physician groups. "If I'm interested in change, I need three things: the will to change; ideas [and] alternatives to the status quo; and the management of change as an ongoing process. With respect to the will, the dues-paying organizations...will always have to play to the middle of the pack. They can't push their members too hard—nor would I, if I were running those organizations. So they have a lot of trouble building the will for change. Most of the large associations, including subspecialty groups, are arguing for further resources for the status quo, and that's not going to get us where we need to go."

There is much more of interest in the interview, including Berwick's views on pay-for-performance and his reservations about the growing trend of employers' shifting all or most of the financial incentives to the patient. But for this essay let's focus on oncology and on two factors emphasized by Berwick above: leadership in health care delivery organizations; and professional organizations as agents of change.

I agree with Berwick that there has been no mainstream effort for improving the quality of care by health systems, hospitals, and health maintenance organizations. There are a few exceptions that have a history of consistent efforts in quality improvement, such as Kaiser Permanente, Virginia Mason Medical Center in Seattle, and Intermountain Healthcare in Utah.

My own observations as a staff member within and a consultant for hospitals and health systems jibe with those made by Berwick. All hospital leaders and trustees pay lip service to quality, but it is rare to find any that have a clue as to the quality of care in their organizations. They accept accreditation by the Joint Commission for Accreditation of Health Care Organizations or the American College of Surgeons, or the local reputation of a surgeon as proof of quality care in their facilities. Or worse, they believe a new

CT scanner or a PET scanner is a sign of high-quality care. Trustees rarely scratch the surface of operations, except for financial issues; too many are chosen to sit on a board of trustees of a non-profit organization because they have money or influence and end up just taking up space.

I can think of several possible reasons for this passivity. First, as Berwick says, trustees may be intimidated by their lack of technical knowledge. Second, they may be intimidated by other trustees who are influential in business or social circles that impact the trustee's personal interests. Third, many believe that their fiduciary responsibility centers on the financial health of the institution and the performance of the chief operating officer (often seeing those two factors as identical), but does not extend to operational issues. (It is true that a board that micromanages an organization is worse than one that is disengaged, but not by much.) But I believe the main reason is ignorance. Most don't know what to ask; they don't know how widely the quality of care varies and the need for continued vigilance to assure the highest quality possible.

What is the solution? I believe that, over time, comprehensive quality measures should be adopted for health care organizations and that the results should be made public. My rationale follows: Asking leaders and trustees in hospitals and health care systems to change their interests and behavior is a losing strategy. They are not prepared or educated for such a task. But trustees will quickly react and demand an explanation when the standing of the institution is publicly revealed to be below par. They all know whether their health care institution is listed, and at what rank, in the annual ranking by *U.S. News and World Report*. In New York State, they all know their institution's ranking in the mortality following cardiac surgery, which is publicized annually by the state. They don't need to know anything about surgery or quality of care to know their institution ranks below average or is not even listed. Consistent public failure would certainly lead the trustees to find new leadership and I guarantee that the new leader would be committed to quality improvement.

But health systems and hospitals are not the only organizations short on effective leaders pushing for higher-quality health care. Congress has done little or nothing—the Kennedy-Frist bill has languished and now has morphed into another version in the Senate, but there is no comparable action in the House. State governors and legislatures have demonstrated little interest, with rare exceptions such as New York and Georgia. And professional associations, with exceptions that include the American College of Cardiology, the Society for Thoracic Surgery, and ASCO, have not been at the forefront of this movement.

My view on the role of physician associations in quality improvement efforts differs in several respects from Berwick's. I agree that professional associations with dues-paying members usually "play to the middle of the pack," thus restricting their ability to initiate change, especially global change. They are built mainly for education and fellowship.

However, there are several factors that can make it possible for associations to improve the quality of care through the membership. First, the goal cannot be to engage and change the practices of *all* members, just those willing to participate, which is likely to be a minority of members. In fact, one must start a program only with the seriously willing to give it the best chance of success. Second, a voluntary program that is not onerous and has physician-led direction will attract not only those with an abiding interest in quality improvement, but those who are competitive and/or curious about how they stand compared to colleagues. Third, there are successful models—the American College of Cardiology, the Society for Thoracic Surgery, and the nascent Quality Oncology Practice Initiative project of ASCO come to mind. They have demonstrated that success breeds success, i.e., once an effort is up and running and has some success, it attracts many other members. And fourth, physicians are beginning to realize that if we don't do this, some bureaucrat will do it to us and we may not like the result.

I believe we should engage in quality improvement efforts because it is the right thing to do, and I have a simple faith that most docs would agree and given a reasonable opportunity, will participate.

In summary, progress in improving the quality of care is much slower than we would like. A lack of will in health care and other centers of power explains much of this lassitude. Professional associations, while crude and unwieldy tools for change, can initiate and sustain quality improvement programs. And despite the clamor of some oncologists for more money that often drowns out other issues, I believe that the majority want to do the right thing for their patients and want to know how they stack up compared to colleagues. That is what we have to build on.

25 January 2006

Reference

[1] Galvin R: Interview: 'A deficiency of will and ambition': A conversation with Donald Berwick. *Health Affairs* Web Exclusive, January 12, 2005

Chapter 3
LIVING WITH DYING

Helping patients face death is a difficult and critically important job for most physicians, especially those who care for patients with high mortality diseases such as cancer. How patients, their families, doctors, and nurses manage this stress has been a lifelong interest of mine. These essays describe how some patients, medical caregivers, and survivors cope with this experience.

LIVING WITH DYING

Dying Patients and the Little Flame

I HAVE BEEN AN ONCOLOGIST FOR FOUR DECADES and dealing with dying patients has been an important part of my professional life. Like every oncologist, I have cared for such patients in the hospital, as outpatients, and by phone when they went home to die. Although most of my patients have been children, I have arranged for older patients to be cared for in a hospice. I am ashamed to admit, however, that in all those years I never visited or made rounds in a hospice.

Why do I feel ashamed? Perhaps beneath all the protective layers of logic and convention, part of me believes I have dumped those patients, abandoned them at their time of greatest emotional and physical need, and I didn't even have the decency or curiosity to find out what kind of place I sent them to. Or perhaps I believe I should have had some personal knowledge of hospices to inform and enrich my clinical portfolio, as well as my leadership and teaching skills. Or maybe I am just older and more thoughtful about end-of-life issues.

Although it is late in my game, I am gratified to report that recently I have made several visits and made rounds at a local inpatient hospice for patients with incurable cancer. My experience was enlightening, heartening, and moving. I knew what to expect in general, of course, but I was unprepared for the atmosphere, the culture, and, dare I say it, the purity of the medical care provided there.

What was it that made such a strong positive impression? First there were the general factors that I would hope to see in any inpatient facility for patients with cancer. But there were features that seemed specific to hospices.

The atmosphere of the two-story facility was welcoming. It was spotlessly clean, spacious, airy, well-lighted and, in a way, cheery. Yes, cheery. Not in a demonstrative or party way, but with an air of quiet friendliness, efficiency, and solicitous care. It was December and there were Christmas decorations in each room and in the halls, gifts and holiday foods for the patients, and on one visit, a quintet played music in the hallways.

The pervasive culture—remarkable respect for the individual patient and of a high level of care—could not have happened by accident. The nursing staff was knowledgeable about palliative medications (far more than me), up to the minute on each patient's pain, other symptoms and bodily functions, and also very tuned in to social and family issues. They and the aides and support staff took outstanding general care of the patients. On every visit, I found all the patients, beds, rooms, and common areas orderly and spotless, and the patients universally comfortable or very nearly so. An experienced local internist made rounds twice weekly and was on call for order changes, but the atmosphere and culture were created and sustained by the onsite staff.

I have worked in great institutions that gave wonderful care, but the atmosphere, culture, and solicitous concern shown for each patient by every member of the staff in the hospice struck me differently, and I wondered why. One answer that came to me has to do with, for want of a better word, the "purity" of care. The care seemed devoid of the many layers of distraction, some necessary, some not, that get between today's caregivers and patients. The sole focus of every activity was the comfort of each patient, with no laboratory tests or diagnostic images, no debilitating therapy, none of the 24/7 bustle and noisy chatter of a typical inpatient unit, and minimal paperwork. Perhaps another factor was that both the prognosis and the goal of care seemed clearly understood and accepted by staff and patient.

But there was something else that seemed to be characteristic of hospice culture. Although the specifics may differ among hospices, that culture was illustrated at the one I visited, Our Lady of Perpetual Help Home in Atlanta. It is one of six owned and operated nationwide by the Dominican Sisters of Hawthorne, a Roman Catholic nursing order.

The order was started in 1900 by the daughter of Nathaniel Hawthorne to care specifically for patients with terminal cancer, regardless of race, creed, or means. The nuns are nurses who lead the staff and personally provide all the nursing care for the female patients; male nurses care for male patients. They accept no payment from patients, no insurance, and no government support; they have no billing department. They prefer to accept no donations from a patient's family, but if pushed will accept no more that $100. Philanthropy sustains them and their work, so the usual economic complexities and compromises of today's health care facilities are not apparent. Dr. Jack Reed, the internist who rounds there, said if he needed such care and could not be at home, it is where he would want to be; I feel exactly the same.

It is a shame that we oncologists fail to use hospices sooner in the course of management and too often, at the cost of proper palliative care, employ futile anti-cancer therapy. The latter often holds out false hope instead of providing more appropriate end-of-life care. Why is it done? It is not easy to tell a patient and family that there is no effective cancer therapy left; and, sad to say, too often economics plays a role. Offering hospice and other end-of-life care is not abandonment or "having no therapy to offer," but another specific kind of therapy; a therapy that for many patients is more appropriate and more humane, to help them live as well as possible while they are dying.

For hospice staffs at Our Lady of Perpetual Help Home and elsewhere, the hospice is like their home both personally and professionally, and the patients are their guests. Their work is a vocation, a calling, and they attract staff members with the same attitude that help sustain that culture. Their vocation is not, as is so often the case in our busy days, buried under the weight of the business of health care, professional ambition, research opportunism, or technical *tours de force*. They can remind us of that little flame of altruistic idealism that burns in all of us in medicine and nursing. Though sometimes dimmed by personal or professional pressures or obscured by overwork or by greed, that flame prevails in each of us ready to remind us that the heart of our vocation makes it special and such a privilege to practice.

10 February 2004

LIVING WITH DYING

Why Work in a Hospice?

EVERY YEAR THE CHRISTMAS SEASON ELICITS IN ME a bit of Ebenezer Scrooge. I am annoyed by the frantic consumerism, the relentless banality of seasonal pop music, and the near burial of the basic Christmas message under the pomp and bustle of the holiday. Eventually, my little Scrooge is converted by the great joy of the family gathering, of receiving Christmas cards with little hand-written notes from old friends, and of hearing the sometimes moving and inspiring carols of hope.

But as I write this several weeks before Christmas, my bit of Scrooge has already been converted. I have just completed interviewing some of the staff at Our Lady of Perpetual Help Home (OLPHH), an inpatient hospice for patients with cancer in Atlanta. I wanted to know what motivated the nurses and aides to choose this work and what were the best and worst parts of the job. So I asked them and here is what they said.

Horace (a certified nurse assistant for 25 years who has worked at OLPHH for 18 years): "I like working here because of the chance to give back compassion and love. This is like home, a brotherhood of co-workers and the Sisters. I find it hard to find the words to describe it. It is home, like a second family. I can't sing or dance, but I sure can take care of people. I get an emotional charge from helping them. The residents here become my friends. Even though their time may be short, I bond with residents and their family. The hardest part of the job is letting go. But I gotta get over it and be strong; if I am weak, I am no good to the resident. The others [coworkers] are my crutches and my foundation in the hard times. You gotta be good here; there are strict regulations to make sure that all residents' needs are met; I like that. The Sisters' [example of] love and compassion is contagious; it hooks you."

Ronnie (a certified nurse assistant who has worked at OLPHH for 17 years): "I like working in a hospice because it helps me better understand my own mortality. It gives a chance to look at yourself deeply and to understand that we are only here for a short time. I like working here [in this hospice] because of the camaraderie, the life experiences, and the religious setup. We are not a company [commercial business], we are a family. It is a rewarding feeling to help people in their final life's journey to the other realm. The hardest part is to "attach but detach." I take good care of all residents, but some leave footprints on your mind, some get next to you. It's hard to let go, but we send them on their way as trouble-free as possible. The best part of the job is helping somebody. On my ward we try to help them have as peaceful, satisfying journey as comfortable as possible."

Charles (a licensed practical nurse who has worked at OLPHH for 3 years):
"I like to give these people a helping hand. This gives me great satisfaction. I also like the religious atmosphere here; it is very conducive for me to play [my] role. The conditions of service here are very good. The hardest part for me is when we get young patients with terminal cancer. It opens your eyes to see people your own age who will die of cancer, not just old people. They are [usually] very scared to face the unknown and we try to help them understand, as much as we know. The best part is that the patients and families are always very appreciative of what we do."

Sister Mary Martha (a registered nurse for 54 years):
"I chose nursing because there were a lot of elderly people in my town who did not get good care. I worked in the operating room for awhile. Then I cared for sick newborns and I thought, "I can't do this for the rest of my life, it is too hard;" it was heartbreaking. I had been thinking about entering a religious order and heard about the Hawthorne Dominican's hospice for patients with cancer in New York and thought, "gee, that sounds good," and planned to visit. (The Hawthorne Dominican order of nuns was founded in the 19th century in New York by the daughter of Nathaniel Hawthorne explicitly for the care of patients terminally ill with cancer.)

"Later, when a spiritual advisor suggested I visit the Hawthorne hospice, I was stunned that he made that suggestion [after I had thought about it earlier], and I thought, "this is where God is calling me." I toured the facility and met a 21-year-old girl there, the same age as me, who had bone cancer and I decided right there that this is what I wanted to do for the rest of my life. It is hard to explain. It was a calling. I didn't realize then that [in addition to giving nursing care] I would help send them off to God. The hardest part for me is dealing with people with mental illnesses; I have always been that way. The best part is taking care of the patients, making them comfortable, taking them out for a stroll—all our houses have nice grounds—and seeing them smile. On Sunday afternoon I [sometimes] would get two ice cream cones, one for the patient and one for me, and wheel them outside and eat and talk. I try to get the best out of my patients, ask them about their childhood (you hear some very funny stories) and help them die happy. I am 75 years old and they want me to retire, but I am not ready. I had a broken leg and after 2 months I said, "I gotta get moving." They don't let me do some things, like take night watch, which I love doing, but I take afternoon watch and help patients and stock shelves. I am just happy doing this work."

Sister Mary Luke (became a registered nurse in 1962, joined the Hawthorne Dominican Order in 1963, and got a B.S. in nursing in 1973):
"I have been in the order for 41 years. I chose the order at 21 because I wanted to do something hard. You know how it is; when you are young you think you can do anything. In those days cancer hospice work didn't have the same status as today and I thought taking care of patients with cancer was kind of heroic. But I found out that it wasn't so hard. Most of the hard decisions have already been made by the patient and the family; they have had all the treatment, so one can focus more on the spiritual and psychological needs and helping the family. It's just amazing how courageous people are. It is a privilege to be with them and their families at their finest hour; it always amazes me how brave people are and how accepting they are. Would I choose this again, knowing what I know? Probably not, because I wouldn't think that I had the strength, so it's a good thing you make those decisions when you are young. I was a young 21 when I entered; a kid. I think the physical part is the only hard part for me, the 7-day week. And sometimes you have to work at night and the next day when you're tired. But that's really the only hard part of this whole life. If I didn't have that I wouldn't have any purgatory [chuckles]. What is the best part of the work? Well, it is a lot of things. It makes my spiritual life easier. And I am never alone; I always have someone to talk to. It is a beautiful life."

Yes, Sister Luke, the way all of you at Our Lady of Perpetual Help Home and other hospices lead it, it is a beautiful life. And thanks to you and your co-workers for the privilege of sharing your example and for reminding me that the Christmas spirit can last 365 days a year, 24/7.

10 January 2005

Intimations of Mortality

ONE OF THE LIFE-CHANGING EXPERIENCES of my fellowship was dealing with children dying of cancer. I struggled with my own emotions and with the search for ways to understand and support the child and family. Experience helped, but I also began to read a wide range of literature on death and dying, which was more limited in the 1960s than today. Part of my search entailed working with a child psychiatrist on a project to interview parents and siblings before and after the death of a child; I saved the recordings and they still have the power to move me. I would often drive home at night thanking God that my three young daughters were healthy.

However, throughout my years of caring for these children, I cannot recall that the experiences made me reflect in any depth on my own mortality. That has come in later years, a product of age, the loss of friends and family, and an enlarging medicine cabinet. For the last decade or more I have been interested in how others view their mortality. I know well the views of religious orthodoxy, but the constriction of dogma rarely leaves sufficient room for the subtlety, contradictions, and mystery inherent in the subject. So I have turned to poets who in older age have addressed their mortality. As one might expect, the varieties of such experience are many, seemingly unique with each person. The following is a sample.

William Wordsworth (1770-1850) is known for the vision in his poetry of the virtues and beauty of nature. He addresses mortality with elegance in "Ode–Intimations of Immortality from Recollections of Early Childhood." The first 50 lines describe in beautiful detail the childhood joy felt in the glory of nature—trees, grass, flowers, wind, birds. And then as he ages in the poem the vision gradually fades, "Whither is fled the visionary gleam? /Where is it now, the glory and the dream? ... At length the Man perceives it die away /And fade into the light of common day."

He later describes the consolations for that loss in his living and in his faith: "What though the radiance which was once so bright /Be now for ever taken from my sight, / Though nothing can bring back the hour /Of splendor in the grass, of glory in the flower; /We will grieve not, rather find /Strength in what remains behind; /In the primal sympathy /Which having been must ever be; /In the soothing thoughts that spring /Out of human suffering; / In the faith that looks through death, /In years that bring the philosophic mind."

Wordsworth concludes with a return to nature and the thoughts it provokes as he considers eventual death: "The clouds that gather round the setting sun /Do take a sober colouring from the eye /That hath kept watch o'er man's mortality; /Another race hath been, and other palms are won, / Thanks to the human heart by which we live, / Thanks to its tenderness, its joys and fears, /To me the meanest flower that blows can give / Thoughts that do often lie too deep for tears." I especially like his use of the sun as an eye that "colours" the clouds and has kept an eternal eye on the mortality of man. And again in the last two lines how a plain and simple flower can provoke such deep thoughts.

From the 19th century, we move to one of the great poets of the 20th. The poetry of Stanley Kunitz (1905-2006) is quite accessible though he often addresses weighty matters. What looks to be a rather simple poem sometimes leaves me groping deeply for its meaning in my own life. My favorite Kunitz book is *Next-to-Last Things: New Poems and Essays*.[1] In addition to wonderful poems, in this thin volume he writes essays on the art and meaning of poetry in a clear and straightforward manner. A blurb on the dustcover may say it best. "The poetry of Stanley Kunitz is not explicitly religious, nor heavily symbolic. Yet it seems to be attended by mysterious presences, by a nearly sacred aura. There are few poets left in our time who seem to carry this bardic authority." And a reviewer states, "Kunitz's poetry sees through to some unknown aspect of his 'beingness' – makes the darkness transparent. [He] is without religion, but preoccupied with God. There is hardly a poem that is not in some way devotional."

The title of the book comes from his poem, "Around Pastor Bonhoeffer," which gives an inkling of his values and thoughts on mortality. Bonhoeffer was a German clergyman who fled Nazi Germany, but returned to protest and give witness against the Nazis; he was later executed by them. "And he forsook the last things, /the dear inviolable mysteries – /Plato's lamp, passed from the hand / of saint to saint–/that he might risk his soul in the streets, /where the things given /are only next to last..."

In "Passing Through – on my seventy-ninth birthday," he is speaking to someone (his wife?) about pushing him into "festive occasions," presumably a birthday party for him; he doesn't much care for them and places that in a larger picture. "Sometimes, you say, I wear /an abstracted look that drives you /up the wall, as though it signified /distress or disaffection. /Don't take it so to heart. /Maybe I enjoy not-being as much /as being who I am. Maybe /it's time for me to practice /growing old. The way I look /at it, I'm passing through a phase; /gradually I'm changing to a word. / Whatever you choose to claim /of me is always yours; /nothing is truly mine /except my name. I only /borrowed this dust."

The 27 short lines (132 words) of "The Image-Maker" should be read in its entirety; it is a jewel of introspection and intimations of mortality.

"A wind passed over my mind, /insidious and cold. /It is a thought, I thought, /but it was only its shadow. /Words came, /on the breath of my sisters, /with a black rustle of wings. /They came with a summons /that followed a blessing. /I could not believe / I too would be punished. /Perhaps it is time to go, /to slip alone, as at a birth, /out of this glowing house /where all my children danced. /Seductive Night! I have stood /at my casement the longest hour, /watching the acid wafer /of the moon slowly dissolving /in a scud of cloud, and heard, /the farthest hidden stars /calling my name. /I listen, but I avert my ears /from Meister Eckhart's warning: /*All things must be forsaken. /God scorns to show Himself among images.*"

Czeslaw Milosz (1911-2004) lived through terrible times and yet his poetry confronts their reality. He loved life and its pleasures, but, especially in his later life, he also struggled to keep his faith and often pondered the tension between the material and the infinite. Perhaps that is why I feel close to him. His book, *Second Space* talks about heaven and hell and how modernity has taken them away from us.[2] "Have we really lost faith in that other space? /Have they vanished forever, both Heaven and Hell? /Without unearthly meadows how to meet salvation? /And where will the damned find suitable quarters? /Let us weep, lament the enormity of the loss. /Let us smear our faces with coal, loosen our hair. /Let us implore that it be returned to us, /That second space."

In his book, *Provinces*,[3] his poem, "A New Province," addresses old age and mortality. "You would like to hear how it is in old age? /Certainly, not much is known about that country /Till we land there ourselves, with no right to return." Thirteen stanzas follow; the fourth: "The course of my dying seems to me amusing. /Weakness of legs, the heart pounding, hard to go uphill. /Myself beside my refractory body. /In the clarity of my mind, as in a mountain nest. /And yet humiliated by difficulty in breathing, / Vanquished by the loss of my hair and my teeth." And in the final stanza, "I would prefer to be able to say: 'I am satiated, /What is given to taste in this life, I have tasted.' / But I am like someone in a window who draws aside a curtain /To look at a feast he does not comprehend."

In the same volume, "Either – Or" (the title recalls the great work of the same title by Søren Kirkegaard) considers whether or not the divinity and resurrection of Jesus is true. If true, we must order our behavior accordingly and we should publicly testify "with words, music, dance and every sign." Or if not: "If what is proclaimed in Christianity is a fiction, /And what we are taught in schools, /In newspapers and TV is true: /That the evolution of life is an accident, /As is an accident the existence of man, /And that his history goes from nowhere to nowhere, /Our duty is to draw conclusions /From our thinking of the innumerable generations /Who lived and died deluding themselves....That our capacity for self-delusion has no limits /And that anybody who believes anything is mistaken. /The only gesture worthy of respect is to complain of our /transience..."

But then he counters. "Not at all! Why either-or? /For centuries men and gods have lived together, /Supplications have been made for health or a successful journey. /Not that one should constantly meditate on who Jesus was. /What can we, ordinary people, know of the Mystery? ... It is better that not everyone is called to priesthood. /Some are for prayers, others for their sins." And he ends the debate thus, "May we not care about what waits us after death /But here on earth look for salvation, /Trying to do good within our limits, /Forgiving the mortals their imperfection. Amen."

These men are trying to come to terms with their aging and mortality and their serious and elegant attempts help me come to terms with mine.

25 September 2006

References
[1] Kunitz S: *Next-to-Last Things: New Poems and Essays*. New York, NY. Atlantic Monthly Press, 1985
[2] Milosz C: *Second Space: New Poems*. New York, NY. Ecco Press, 2004
[3] Milosz C: *Provinces: Poems 1987-1991*. New York, NY. Ecco Press, 1993

A Poet Faces Cancer

———→⊃●⊂———

IT WOULD NOT BE SURPRISING that an oncologist might think about facing death more than, say, a dermatologist or a plumber. That said, I believe I think about it more than most, or at least I express it more; recent essays have addressed the struggle of surviving the death of a loved one and of caring for patients terminally ill with cancer in a hospice. I am not certain why this is so. Caring for so many dying children and their families early in my career certainly played a role. A lifelong curiosity about the "big questions" of living and dying usually addressed by philosophers, scientists, and theologians—Why am I here? Where am I going? How do I live a "good" life? How will I face the death of a loved one or myself?—naturally has also kept those thoughts popping in and out of my consciousness.

People often have strongly held beliefs concerning life after death. Most scientists and secularists believe death is the end with no afterlife; most of those with religious faith believe that there is an afterlife, though exactly what that entails varies widely among and even within religious faiths; philosophers also don't have a clue. But none of them has convincing and useful advice for how we are to face our own death.

Artists, and especially poets, may come closest to providing a glimpse of living with and facing death. Their skills somehow have the power, on occasion, to touch us deeper than the others. They do this by subtlety and indirection, by gently immersing us deeper and deeper into their thoughts and feelings. Before we know it, we see a dim light of understanding, not from logic or dogma or data, but by osmosis from the poet. Not all who read such a poem or see such a painting will experience that enlightenment, but when it happens it is not easily forgotten.

I read such a poem recently by Tony Hoagland.[1] I have since re-read it many times with the same enlightening effect. The poet does not describe death or its sequelae, but he describes facing (or how he would face) death from cancer. I reproduce it here in its entirety with permission of the author. I cannot guarantee your reaction will be like mine. But at the very least, this accessible, lovely poem should be enjoyable; it is certainly relevant to our work.

Barton Springs

Oh life, how I loved your cold spring mornings
of putting my stuff in the green gym-bag
and crossing wet grass to the southeast gate
to push my crumpled dollar through the slot.

When I get my allotted case of cancer,
let me swim ten more times at Barton Springs,
in the outdoor pool at 6am, in the cold water
with the geezers and jocks.

With my head bald from radiation
and my chemotherapeutic weight loss
I will be sleek as a cheetah
–and I will not complain about life's

pedestrian hypocrisies,
I will not consider death a contractual violation.
Let my cancer be the slow-growing kind
so I will have all the time I need

to backstroke over the rocks and little fishes,
looking upward through my bronze-tinted goggles
into the vaults and rafters of the oaks,
as the crows exchange their morning gossip

in the pale mutations of early light.
It was worth death to see you through these optic nerves,
to feel breeze through the fur on my arms
to be chilled and stirred in your mortal martini.

In documents elsewhere I have already recorded
my complaints in some painstaking detail.
Now, because all things are joyful near water,
There just might be time to catch up on praise.

Reprinted with permission of Tony Hoagland

10 August 2007

Reference

[1] Hoagland T: Barton Springs. *Poetry* 190:247, 2007

My Mother

SIX DAYS AGO I RECEIVED A CALL that my mother had been hospitalized because of diarrhea and vomiting. My mother will be 93 years old in November and for years she has been hospitalized every few months for a couple of days for what I have come to call her "tune-ups." She has insulin-dependent diabetes, hypertension, borderline congestive heart failure, borderline renal function, fluctuating liver function tests, and chronic back pain from severe osteoarthritis. None of this is new. Her physicians have done an amazing job over many years of balancing the treatment of her various problems. The suburban Chicago community she lives in provides a visiting nurse and a physician who makes occasional house calls when the nurse asks. Her hospitalizations usually are due to early pulmonary edema or a respiratory infection. But none of this says anything specific about my mother as a person, which is at the heart of this story.

My mother arrived in Chicago from the mountains of rural Sicily in 1931 with her mother and brother. She was 17 years old. Her father was a barber who had come years earlier to make the money to send for his family. My grandfather did not drive, so he asked one of his customers, a taxicab driver, to go with him to the railroad station to bring his family home. The taxicab driver was my father, himself an immigrant who had arrived in the United States 10 years earlier; they were married 3 years later and I was born 4 years later. They settled on the west side of Chicago and worked hard to raise four children and make a loving and happy household.

With some intravenous fluids, my mother's symptoms resolved. However, because she had some abdominal soreness, they did a CT scan of her abdomen. They found a suspicious mass and an ultrasound exam confirmed that she had a 3.5 cm solid mass in the head of the pancreas with some ductal dilation. The mass apparently had caused no symptoms and was an incidental finding. Before I learned of this, her physician had given her the news and said she would need surgery. She flatly refused and said she wanted to go home. When I talked to her she remained steadfast. She would have no surgery and no further tests.

Now I can hear all the oncologists out there saying that at least she needs a biopsy because it could be a benign tumor, though that is unlikely. And what about a stent to prevent jaundice when the time comes? In order to understand my mother's position, you will need further information.

First, there are two key facts: 1) all of her mental faculties are as sharp as ever; 2) she is fiercely independent. Despite her physical problems, she continues to live alone in an apartment about 20 minutes from my sister. She has difficulty walking and sleeps fitfully, but has declined to move to an assisted living facility, despite many attempts by my sister and me over the past 15 years. Her response has been, "I'm not going to no nursing home!" But Mom, we persist, it is not a nursing home, etc., etc. "They are all nursing homes," she retorts. Then we offered to build an addition onto my sister's house for her or to have her leave Chicago and move in with us. She declined both for a variety of reasons, none of which was the central reason, which will become clear to you as it finally did to me.

Second, for her age, medical condition, and environment, she has remarkable control of her life and has remained largely independent. She has friends in her apartment building who shop for her groceries, pick up her prescriptions, take out her garbage, and visit with her periodically. A woman comes to clean the house, my sister drops in to bring her food, and a local dentist offered to refit her dentures with a few house calls (home-made assisted living?). She still cooks a little and if she chooses not to, she puts a Lean Cuisine frozen dinner in the microwave. She controls her own heat and air conditioning. She tests her blood sugar, injects her own insulin, and takes her own medicine. And she attends Mass (via television) every day and keeps up with the news.

And finally, while my mother is physically frail, she has an iron will that has occasionally created sparks with her family, but has gotten her through hard times and personal tragedy. She endured a parent's nightmare twice: she has buried two of her four children, a baby boy who died of croup in the 1940s and an adult daughter who died of surgical complications. Her husband—my father—died in 1968 so she has been a widow for almost 40 years. She gets lonely at times, but doesn't want anyone to stay too long because entertaining takes effort and it can disrupt a routine that is comfortable. The routine allows her to pace herself in expending energy, talk to her kids, grandkids, and great-grandkids on the phone, see her programs on TV, and take care of her medical and other personal needs.

So it gradually became clear over the years that on my mother's list of values, maintaining control and independence trumps everything else. That has been her strength. That is why she won't go to a "nursing home," that's why she won't move in with my sister or me, that's why she won't have major surgery. Without asking my opinion, she believes that she would never fully recover from major surgery and would be totally dependent, probably for the rest of her life. Without asking my opinion, she believes the prognosis is poor with or without treatment and that if one opts for no treatment, there is no reason to go through a bunch of uncomfortable tests. She may not be educated, but she certainly isn't stupid.

So what now? She has no symptoms attributable to the tumor yet. We have arranged to have a woman stay with her for several hours each day but, as before, she doesn't want anyone for longer. I have contacted my Chicago pals about hospice services and have talked to several social workers there. I would like to have her move in with me, but I am certain she will not leave an environment she has lived in for 75 years. So we will all wait. Her family will visit with her often. And we will let this woman use her strength to guide us in helping her as best we can.

The prospect of losing a parent is never easy; 38 years after his death I still think of and miss my father every day. I think a lot about how hard she and my father worked to raise us and send us to school, the sacrifices they made, and the warmth and love that pervaded our household.

She asked me a few days ago, "Will this be long?" I said, "I don't know, Mom." And then she said, "Do we want to know?" That caught me off guard and I mumbled something about having no biopsy and insufficient information. And what did she mean by "we"? She is still in control and her son is no match for her. She has had a full and meaningful life and, because we love her and owe her so much, we will help her live out the rest of her life – her way.

25 October 2006

LIVING WITH DYING

My Mother – Final Act

MY MOTHER DIED PEACEFULLY LAST NIGHT. It had been only three 3 weeks since the diagnosis of pancreatic cancer. It has been a memorable 3 weeks not because of sadness, pain, and anguish, but because of the joy of the family celebrating her long and eventful life with her. She directed the action in typical fashion from the time of diagnosis until the last day.

First, she declined any therapy or further diagnostic tests and insisted on going home from the hospital. The first week home was a happy one for her as she made preparations. She had no symptoms until the end of the week when she became jaundiced, which I had alerted her and my sister to look for. She had the home health nurse take away the monitoring equipment (cardiac pacemaker). When I visited with her the next weekend, I told her she did not need to take any of her medications, which made her very happy. I then told her she didn't even need to take her insulin or test her blood sugar anymore; she was ecstatic. This worried my sister, "What will happen?" I said nothing would happen except she might pee more.

Her home health doctor had visited just before we arrived and because the jaundice was causing some itching, he had suggested that a stent be put in via endoscope. She said she would talk to me about it and when I arrived she said, "I will do whatever you say." I knew this was not true, unless my advice happened to agree with her decision, but I called Dr. Chiang (a saint who cared for her for years) and got the details of what would be involved. I then explained to my mother and sister without editorial comment that she would go to the hospital, have anesthesia, have a tube inserted and that they might need to make small cuts to enlarge the orifice, etc. She said, "Why go through all that for some itching? I have had bad back pain every day for years (osteoarthritis); this is nothing." I told her that I agreed with her decision, which made her happy. So we got various forms of Benadryl lotion and pills to control the itching, and they worked pretty well.

My sister and her husband, my wife and I spent the whole day with her discussing her wishes. She was laser-focused on who would get her furniture. She offered it to all of us, knowing we would decline. But following her protocol of tradition, she then wanted to know if any of our kids (her seven grandchildren) wanted any of the furniture, and insisted we call and find out, which we did. All declined except one niece who wanted to restore the "antique" bedroom furniture and another niece who wanted the cedar chest. After the family had its chance, she decided who would get the rest among long-standing neighbors and friends.

I had told my mother she could now eat anything she wanted. She ate ice cream, which she loved but hadn't eaten because of her diabetes, and yogurt every day until the last few days. As I was leaving that evening to sleep at my sister's house, she said, "Don't forget to bring something for lunch tomorrow." I asked what she wanted and she said, "Kentucky Fried Chicken...dark meat."

Before we left, she asked (ordered?) that her four great-grandchildren that lived nearby come to her apartment the next day. She wanted them to open the two piggy banks she had and divide the coins there in front of her. Needless to say, they came the next day. Finding the piggy banks was a challenge; her directions (or memory) were not very clear. We sifted through tons (not much of an exaggeration) of old papers, utility bills, greeting cards, clothing, religious artifacts, etc., and finally located them. The kids (8 to 12 years old) had a ball helping us look and dutifully sat on the floor in front of her and sorted and distributed the coins. My mother was very happy. She had taken care of the furniture and the coins and she said, "The rest is junk," meaning she didn't care what we did with it.

It was a great weekend for her and for us. She did pretty well for a few days but her appetite declined steadily and she said she was tired. We had arranged for home hospice care. When I returned a few days later, she had declined noticeably and was sleeping a great deal without medications. However, when aroused her memory and mind were as sharp as ever, which remained true until the last 24 hours. I spent three days with her and before returning home to take care of some business, I spoke with her and told her I was leaving but would be back. Two hours after I arrived home from the airport, I got a call that she had died peacefully.

We will have a traditional wake and she will be buried next to her husband and with her baby son who died in 1943, just as she had planned for years.

In another age, my mother would have been a leader in business. She was bright beyond her meager education. She had the kind of independence, strength of will, and confidence in her judgments that makes good leaders. I see a bit of her better traits in me, my sisters, and my daughters, and I am grateful for that.

10 November 2006

LIVING WITH DYING

Mourning and Grieving For Chris

WHEN BAD THINGS HAPPEN IN OUR LIVES, we deal with them in different ways: we may face the consequences and try to mitigate them; try to hide them with distractions; blame someone or something for the misfortune; try to forget, with or without chemical help; or find consolation in a remembrance. But when the bad thing is the death of a loved one, our main response is to grieve and mourn the loss. My experiences as a pediatric oncologist—and with life in general—have taught me that grief and mourning differ widely in depth, duration, and effect. In a sense, depending on the circumstances, we see things through a glass that has different colors and shades that influence the emotional impact.

As much as I can recall, mourning the death of my infant brother when I was 7 years old was largely from seeing and feeling the profound grief of my devastated parents. Although I grieve my mother's death two months ago at age 92, she had pancreatic cancer, chose to have no therapy, and enjoyed several weeks of family around her celebrating her life. She said, "I don't want any sadness around here; I am in no hurry, but I am ready to go." She died peacefully in her sleep. My father's death in 1968 at the age of 64 (I was 32) has affected me most profoundly; I think of him and grieve the loss almost every day. Many of my patients died of leukemia in the early years of my career, infants to teenagers. I mourned the loss, especially the pain suffered by their parents, but I was working at finding better treatment for others like them; this seemed to help me emotionally.

The latest mourning in my life has affected me deeply, perhaps because of the person and the circumstances. First, here is part of the obituary that appeared in the Richmond, Virginia newspaper.

Dr. Christopher E. Desch, 51, of Richmond, National Medical Director of the National Comprehensive Cancer Network, died Sunday Dec. 10, 2006, when the private plane he was piloting crashed due to engine failure near Charlottesville. Chris earned his undergraduate degree in 1977 from Ohio State University, where he received his Doctor of Medicine degree, summa cum laude, in 1981. He started his VCU career in 1988 following a residency in internal medicine at the University of Rochester from 1981 to 1984. He was the Medical Chief Resident from 1984 to 1985. He completed a fellowship in Hematology and Oncology at the University of Washington from 1985 to 1988. He was board-certified in Internal Medicine, Oncology and Hematology and was a Fellow of the American College of Physicians. Chris was a parishioner at the Cathedral of the Sacred Heart. He was a subscriber and donor to the Barksdale Theatre. He was a member of the Country Club of Virginia and the Wingnuts Flying Club. He loved his family, his friends, his patients and their families, as well as golf, dancing, poetry, Starbucks coffee, bright ties, wild socks, food, and of course, flying. He was an enthusiastic and loyal Buckeye fan. Chris is preceded in death by his father John J. "Jack" Desch. He is survived by his wife, Roxanne Cherry, and their son, John Tobias "Toby" Desch; his mother, Geraldine O. Desch, of Dayton, a sister and four brothers. The family requests all memorials be sent to the Evans Scholars Foundation, 1 Briar Road, Golf, Illinois, 60029. The memorials will endow in name the Doctor Christopher E. Desch Room at the new Scholarship House being built at the Ohio State University. Without the support from this national scholarship organization none of his education, and therefore his work, would have been possible.

Those are the facts, but Chris was a good friend and close colleague. His death is devastating to me personally, a great loss for our profession and, especially, a terrible loss for his wife, Roxanne and his son, Toby. He was one of the founding volunteer docs of the Quality Oncology Practice Initiative (QOPI) for the American Society of Clinical Oncology (ASCO), which is how I got to know him well and work with him for the past several years. He was smart, kind, funny, and perceptive. He was always trying to do the right thing and to make things clearer and easier for us, which, I am confident, is how he was with his patients, staff. and other colleagues. It is just the way he was, deep down in his heart. He inspired us to press on when things were rocky; he provided the unique perspective of one who was both an academic and community oncologist. The Steering Committee of QOPI – Chris, Mike Neuss, Peter Eisenberg, Joe Jacobson, Kristen McNiff, and I ~ met often by e-mail and conference calls over the years; that has been one of the best professional and personal relationships I have ever had.

When I got the news by e-mail from Kris McNiff, I responded, "Thanks, Kris. I can imagine it hasn't been easy for the family to focus on the arrangements. We in oncology think we appreciate how evanescent life can be, but only when it hits a loved one do we feel it deep down." Later, in an e-mail exchange with Mike Neuss, he wrote in response to my comment, "This is too true, and the experience of re-learning that you can't deal with a friend's death the way we deal with a patient's death is important and perhaps worth developing in a reflection on Chris's life. Deb Schrag [another colleague] and I were talking about it, and we acknowledged that we regularly walk from a room having pronounced the death of one patient into the neighboring room and begin joking with the next patient who's trusting us to be their doctor, and then we get busy with other patients and give little thought to either of them through the rest of the day. And the reason we were talking about it is because we were both sort of lost and confused about why we were feeling so differently about Chris's death (in contrast to that of the many dying patients we've cared for). We both rationally understand that a life is a life and any death a tragedy for someone, but we were (and are) finding it difficult to just keep moving right now."

Chris died two days after I had surgery so flying to Richmond for the funeral was risky. I called his wife Roxanne to express my feelings and she told me not to worry about coming, "Hearing your voice is enough; Chris would probably have said that you guys should go golfing instead." I was told the church was packed—standing room only—with family, friends, colleagues, and patients, and that the service and the sentiments expressed to the crowd by his 19-year-old son, Toby, were beautiful and memorable.

I shall regret forever not attending Chris's funeral, not because of him or Roxanne and his family, but for me. I just felt a need to mourn there in person, a more satisfying way of paying homage to a caring doctor, wonderful colleague, and joyful friend. But the phone call and this essay must suffice. Bon voyage, Chris; you will always be in our hearts.

25 January 2007

Death and Grieving Survivors

I DIDN'T THINK VERY DEEPLY ABOUT DEATH and grief until my fellowship years in pediatric hematology-oncology.

While growing up, members of my extended family had died and I had witnessed grieving by relatives, but I cannot say that I had more than a superficial understanding of their grief. In our Italian-American culture at that time, wakes were major events and my sisters and I always went with our parents. Wakes lasted 3 nights and many friends and relatives attended more than one night. Women in the immediate family of the deceased wore black and most men wore suits and black ties. There were so many flowers that the smell sometimes made me sick. Upon arriving, we went up to see the body of the deceased and knelt and said a prayer (we kids just stared at the body). Then we would visit the decedent's close relatives, who sat near the casket, to express our condolences; the women always had a forlorn look and held a wet handkerchief. My mother and father then sat and chatted with friends, catching up on the news since the last wedding or funeral. We kids looked for something to do outside the chapel; we hung around with cousins and looked for where the food and drink was kept.

Sometimes we went to the burial in the long procession of cars from the church to the cemetery. At graveside, there often was loud wailing by the wife or mother of the deceased. As the casket was lowered into the grave, I recall there was sometimes a bit of suspenseful drama with quiet whispers that "she might try to jump in with him." We kids always paid close attention, but I never saw anyone do it.

What I learned as a child and teenager from these experiences was that people died, relatives of the deceased were very sad and they cried a lot, and that there was an important ritual to be performed that we were a part of, which for us ended at the cemetery. And if the deceased was a married man, his widow often wore black for an entire year, and sometimes longer. I felt sadness when I was with those grieving, but the feeling was fleeting.

Except for my poorly understood glimpse of my parents' grief at the death from croup of my 9-month-old brother when I was 6, I had little appreciation of the impact of grief. Even when I was a medical student and then an internal medicine resident dealing with patients dying in the hospital, the grief of survivors often was witnessed only briefly or not at all; usually we barely knew the family. I had only a vague and incomplete notion of what impact grief would have on survivors the next day, much less during the coming year and beyond.

My awakening came soon after starting my fellowship. I now had continuous and far greater responsibility. I saw my patients at every outpatient visit and every day they were hospitalized. At every visit I also saw a parent, usually the mother or both mother and father, so a closeness to the patient and family often developed. We pediatricians often complain that the medical establishment too often looks upon children as little adults. One reason for this complaint is that the relationship of doctor and nurse with the patient is enriched and complicated by the essential role and consistent presence and of the parents and family. A second reason is that the patients are babies and children and unique skills and patience are needed to earn their trust. And once trust is established, a special bond of affection and even love is often formed.

And in those early years of the chemotherapy era, virtually all of my patients died. I was confronted with the ineffable and inconsolable sadness and grief of the parents and family. I had two babies of my own and couldn't imagine losing them, much less how I could possibly manage if I did.

I began to wonder how I could help those families, whether there was anything I could do before or after the death of a child. There was always sympathy, but not much help from my colleagues. At that time, and it is probably largely true today, one was expected to suck it up, deal with it, and move on. But I found it difficult to move on. So I began to read everything I could find about death and dying and grief. Most of what I found was in a philosophical or religious vein; that was interesting, but wasn't much help for what I wanted. Then I got lucky.

I went to see the chair of psychiatry and explained my interest. He introduced me to a child psychiatrist, Dr. Ed Futterman, who became intrigued by it. He suggested that we explore family grief after the death of a child by interviewing them. For me this was uncharted waters; luckily he was a very skilled interviewer of adults as well as children. My relationship with most families was good so they agreed to talk to us about the painful experience. We usually interviewed families, siblings as well as parents individually, months after the child died. We made recordings of some of these interviews with their permission and I still have some of them.

The experience was life-changing for me. All family members were still grieving, but the depth and manifestations were quite varied. Anger aimed at God or themselves or (indirectly) at us was common. In one case a mother was convinced that the child got leukemia because she wasn't a good housekeeper and that some infectious agent from dirty dishes caused the disease; no amount of trying to explain it away with science had any effect.

But the interview I remember best was with a pre-school sibling close in age to the deceased child. I was not present; Futterman believed, and I agreed, that this was a delicate matter and he needed to do it without me or the parents. Later, we listened to the tape together. I was amazed at Futterman's tact and skill and astonished at what this 3-year-old boy knew and expressed. When asked what he thought would happen to Robby after he got leukemia, he said, "he gonna die." How did he learn this? He overheard other kids talking. Futterman asked him about how his parents acted after Robby got leukemia. He said, in effect, that they spent more time with Robby, that they loved Robby but didn't love him. Even this small sample gave us an eye-opening taste of the lasting and sometimes devastating impact of grief on the whole family.

After I finished my fellowship and went to St. Jude, my interest in this issue continued. An invited speaker, Dr. Elizabeth Kübler-Ross, had begun writing about death and dying and was a proponent of open discussion and a better understanding of the psychological phases of death and grief. Dr. Myron Karon, who was at the National Cancer Institute, wrote a paper about the lack of openness and candor by the doctors, nurses, and parents with patients. No one even told children the name of their disease. Of course they knew, he said. Just like the little boy we interviewed, there are many ways to hear it. But the silence prevented candid discussion and created a wall between parents and child, making the subsequent grief even worse.

After all the reading I have done, for me the best book on grief is a recent one. *The Year of Magical Thinking* by Joan Didion is a wonder[1] Ms Didion describes the impact of the sudden death at the dinner table of her husband of 40 years, the famous writer John Gregory Dunne. She talks about trying to make sense of it, trying to relive it, and of not changing anything in the house in case he came back. This, and all the other magical thinking that this intelligent, thoughtful woman went through, makes for a stunning and truly enlightening reading experience. Her skills as a professional writer make the book the deepest, most impressive, and most informative description of grief I have seen.

I believe Didion's book should be required reading for all oncology trainees and for anyone who wants to understand the potential impact of the death of oneself or of a loved one. Because of it, after all these years I finally have a small handle on the meaning of grief.

25 June 2007

Reference

[1] Didion J: *The Year of Magical Thinking*. New York, NY. Alfred A. Knopf, 2006.

Albert and Samuel

A RECENT E-MAIL FROM SISTER EDWIN asked if I could come down to Our Lady of Perpetual Help Home to see two new patients. Three of us volunteer to cover on weekends because the regular doctor visits only on Monday and Thursday. By law, admissions must be seen by a physician within 48 hours and if we can't go, they can't admit. Our Lady is a residential hospice for patients terminally ill with cancer who pay nothing; it has no billing department. Almost all patients are poor and have no one who can care for them. The experience today would prove touching in unexpected ways.

I drove down to Our Lady and reviewed the charts of both patients. Both had been referred from Grady Memorial Hospital, Atlanta's large county hospital that provides care mostly for poorer African-Americans.

Albert is a 75-year-old African-American man who had been in reasonably good health and lived independently. He had worked for the railroad and was a military veteran. His first symptom was difficulty swallowing beginning 2 months ago. He was seen at the Veterans Administration hospital outpatient clinic where a contrast study showed a large mass in the esophagus. He did not return there. A few weeks later, his symptoms had worsened. He developed hoarseness and an inability to swallow even his saliva, so he went to Grady because it "was closer." His weight had fallen from 175 to 115 pounds and he was dehydrated so they began intravenous fluids with dietary supplements. He was told he had cancer and he refused further diagnostic tests, so he was referred to Our Lady.

He was very thin, spoke with difficulty because of hoarseness, and constantly coughed up saliva and phlegm. He said he had no pain and except for the copious oral phlegm, was comfortable. The rest of the physical exam was not remarkable, but also was irrelevant. He had declined cancer therapy and had come to Our Lady to die.

Samuel is a 61-year-old African-American man with no known family. He was found to have a squamous carcinoma at the base of the tongue in November 2005. He apparently had some limited therapy in his home town. But the tumor continued to grow obstructing his trachea and pharynx, so he required both a tracheostomy and a percutaneous gastrostomy feeding tube. He had not seen a physician for over a year when he was admitted to Grady with weight loss, dehydration, and electrolyte imbalance. He was found to have multiple metastases in the lungs, abdomen, liver, and bones. He was told the prognosis and was referred to Our Lady.

These men are typical of most of the patients I have seen at Our Lady. They are from the backwater of our society. They are not only financially poor, but they have non-existent or severely stretched domestic support systems. Outside the mainstream of medical care, they often show up with far advanced disease. We could discuss endlessly why this is the case, whose "fault" it is, why society averts its eyes, and what should be done about it. But it was not indignation that I felt.

On the way home my eyes welled up and I asked myself why I was so moved this time. Even if there are caring family members, in a sense these men are a bit like the homeless; they are so alone. And I understood once again that these men are me; they are all of us. Whatever my social rank and despite access to the best of care, it could just as easily have been me in that bed.

But I was moved mainly because I realized that without words the staff at Our Lady had said to the men: "No one else either can or wants to take care of you; we can and we do. No one else knows what to do for you; we do. Come to us and you will not be alone for the rest of your days. We will care for you as one of our own, simply because you are a member of our human family."

10 May 2007

Chapter 4

BEING A DOCTOR

I love being a doctor and being with doctors. How doctors carry out their responsibilities and face the ever changing public and private challenges to their practices is of great interest to me. I describe in these essays some of those challenges as well as exemplary physicians, past and present.

The Rise and Fall of Trust in the Medical Profession

THE SEEMING INABILITY OF THE MEDICAL PROFESSION to influence legislation in the past few years has made me wonder why. When I was growing up just before and after the Second World War, the medical profession was a respected spokesman for the public on health issues. Family doctors often were revered members of the community. Our family went to the same doctor for as long as I can remember; he cared for my mother for 50 years. But today a majority of Americans do not trust the medical profession to run the health system, control health care reforms, or to provide the best solutions for problems of American medicine. What happened between then and now?

In the eyes of those who decide policy, business leaders, and the public, the stature of the medical profession went through a long rise and fall during the 20th century. Mark Schlesinger of Yale University, in an article in the *Milbank Quarterly*, examined in detail this phenomenon (which applied to other professions, as well).[1] He develops potential explanations for it and then examines available data to test those ideas. Unless stated otherwise, the authors cited are referenced in Schlesinger's article.

During most of the 19th century the medical profession suffered low esteem. But bolstered by scientific advances and the reform of medical schools, the early decades of the 20th century saw traditional medicine evolve from an occupation with a mixed reputation and little political influence into one that would "dominate both policy and lay perceptions of health problems" (Freidson). By the middle of the 20th century, the medical profession could virtually dictate most state-level policymaking involving health and could strongly influence federal policy.

However, this rise in influence peaked after World War Two and then began to falter. In my view, the turning point was in the 1960s, a time of general rebellion and distrust of political and professional authority. The American Medical Association (AMA) vigorously fought the establishment of Medicare in 1965. (Years earlier it had also fought the universal vaccination of children by nurses in schools and health departments.) This approach helped erode the profession's stature as an agent for the public interest.

In the 1970s, Barber wrote, "Everywhere in the United States the professions have reached new heights of social power and prestige...yet everywhere they are also in trouble, criticized for their selfishness, their public irresponsibility, their lack of effective self-control, and their resistance to requests for more lay participation in the vital decisions professionals make affecting laymen."

By the 1980s, commentators that included leaders of the medical profession were warning of the "deprofessionalization" of American medicine, that is, the loss of both autonomy and authority (the latter meaning the ability to shape public policy, i.e., to influence "elite decision makers"). In effect, medicine was becoming more like a trade than a profession. Serial public opinion surveys from 1965-2000 show a slow, steady decline of public confidence in the medical profession.

By the end of the 20th century public confidence in the medical profession had declined substantially and the almost routine deference of policy makers to the profession had disappeared. This long arc of rise and fall has been described by Elliott Krause as the "fall of a giant." Schlesinger offers four potential explanations for this change.

Doubts about professional efficacy

In recent decades doubts have been fueled by public awareness of errors in medical judgment, the widespread variation in the prevalence of procedures, unfulfilled promises of over-hyped treatments, and widely recommended treatments that prove unnecessary or even dangerous, such as, super-radical mastectomy, Vioxx, post-menopausal hormone therapy, and conflicting advice on healthy diets. While scientific promise has been hailed and doctors have enjoyed the resulting legitimacy and authority, to an extent its failure is also blamed on doctors. I cannot count how often taxi drivers or other casual acquaintances ask, on learning I am an oncologist, "When will they find a cure for cancer, doc?" This leads to doubts about investments in medical care and research.

Questions about professional agency

Historically, part of the authority and trust awarded the medical profession was the belief that professionals will act as reliable agents that subordinate their own self-interest to the client's well-being. This altruistic orientation is tested by the tension between what is best for an individual patient and for society as a whole. Physicians face a double bind when these two admirable goals conflict, as in cost containment of medical care. The medical profession has done a poor job of articulating a clear principle for balancing those needs. The growth of commercial relationships of physicians with pharmaceutical and medical instrument companies, physician advertising, and the growth of America's market-oriented medical system have eroded the trust in physicians' motives.

The rise of countervailing authority

Authority over medical care that was largely vested in the medical profession in the first half of the 20th century has been challenged by the greater role of government, employers and insurance plans, and the empowerment of individual consumers. Schlesinger believes employers and consumers "pose the greatest threats to the authority of the American medical profession." Business leaders have been highly critical of the medical profession, often portraying doctors as the culprits of health cost inflation. (I guess a market economy is a good thing only if it works in your own favor.) The internet, patient advocacy groups, and aggressive advertising have by turns informed (or misinformed) the public and in the process reduced the influence of the medical profession.

The violation of professional boundaries

As indicated earlier, the medical profession has been weakened by overtly political activities, such as opposition to Medicare by the AMA in the face of strong public support, so "People still trusted their own doctors...but they began to view the medical profession as a whole as greedy and heartless" (Krause).

Schlesinger tested these hypotheses in 1995 by a study using interviews and surveys of both the general public and congressional staffers. In one study, questions measured respondents' support for the authority of the medical profession. A sample follows.

In response to, "The best solutions to problems of American medicine come from relying on those who provide health services," 29% of the general public and 18% of the political elites agreed. To, "The health care system would work better if doctors had full control over the system," only 18% of the general public and 2% of the political elite agreed (the interviews occurred not long after the proposal and failure of the Clinton health plan). "Health care reform should be physician-run instead of other alternatives," was supported by 37% of the general public and 30% of the political elite. "Medical care should be allocated by physician-run groups" was supported by 48% of the public and 22% of the political elite. Thus, there was support for some control of the allocation of resources by physicians, but not full control of policy or reform.

What are we to make of this historical trend?

That the "power elite" in politics and business mistrusts doctors more than the general public is not surprising since there will always be struggles when very large amounts of money and substantial authority is at stake. I for one would not attribute this antipathy to a substantially greater commitment to the public interest among business and political leaders.

Also, these same trends have been observed in many professions. The acts of hubris (and self-interest over public interest) of organized medicine in the mid-20th century seem especially contemptible now, but the esteem of lawyers, politicians, and other professionals has suffered as well. Thus, these trends are due in part to a continuation of the declining respect for all authority that began in the 1950s and was fueled by the civil rights movement and Vietnam War. The information explosion, prosperity, vast internal migration, and other secular trends have contributed to these changes.

Though the public's attitude toward individual doctors has followed a similar downward trend, it has been less severe and fluctuates more widely. This is due to the impact of individual and community circumstances and the powerful inclination to trust in one's own doctor. It is not unusual for patients to have complete faith in their own doctors, but mistrust the profession as a whole.

I must admit that I am not unhappy to see the decline in political and policy influence of the medical profession to its current level. I fear great unilateral secular power in the hands of any group. History is replete with examples of political leaders, churches, military, and professional organizations becoming intoxicated with their power and losing their way. Lord Acton said "Power corrupts and absolute power corrupts absolutely." With great power, organizations tend to forget who they are meant to serve and their main reasons for being.

The medical profession is still very influential today, certainly enough to be heard in public discourse. The more it acts in the public interest, even at the sacrifice of its own self-interest, the more people will listen and trust.

25 April 2007

Reference
[1] Schlesinger M: A loss of faith: The sources of reduced political legitimacy for the American medical profession. *Milbank Quarterly* 80: 185-235, 2002

BEING A DOCTOR

Oncologists Who Make Me Proud to Be One

A FRIEND AND COLLEAGUE RECENTLY DESCRIBED an oncology practice he has dealt with as follows:

> I am sure it is one of the best places in the country to get chemotherapy treatment and have cancer. They have some of the best nurses I've seen. One was voted Oncology Nurse of the Year by the ONS [Oncology Nursing Society] about 8-10 years ago. They know where all the patients live [and] what their means are. They deliver food and clothing around Christmas to the poorest ones. They have finagled all sorts of behind the scenes [legal] ways for patients to get the medicines they need. They have regular support groups, educational sessions, programs...about different cancers—all much more than any practice I've encountered in bigger cities. A palliative care unit started this summer.

This description would be remarkable enough—and any practice would be delighted to receive such kudos from an experienced and keen-eyed oncologist—except for one thing: the practice he described is in a rural area and has no full-time oncologist. An oncologist visits for one day three to four times a month.

How can this be? Has my colleague portrayed the practice from an emotional point of view out of his friendship with the staff there? If he is accurate, how can such a structure work so well?

The colleague who told me this is Dr. Chris Desch, a medical oncologist in Richmond, Virginia.[†] In 1988, one of his first jobs after fellowship training at the Massey Cancer Center of the Medical College of Virginia (MCV) in Richmond, now Virginia Commonwealth University (VCU), was to develop a "reach out" program for oncologically underserved areas within a 100-mile radius of Richmond. Desch and his colleague, Dr. Tom Smith, gradually built the program to help patients and communities in the area, but also with an academic component so they could learn from and report on their efforts. Here is a description of the rationale for the program from a paper written by Desch.

[†] Deceased (see "Mourning and Grieving for Chris" pp 97-99)

The Rural Cancer Outreach Program (RCOP) is an effort to bring the best available cancer treatment and prevention to rural Virginia. Rural patients and physicians sensed a need for cancer services based on the perceived prevalence of cancer, the reluctance of patients to travel to the urban treatment centers, and the inability of some to pay for their care. Physicians related several experiences of patients refusing curative or palliative therapy because of the distance. Administrators perceived a need for the hospital to be more responsive to the community, to create a linkage with a prestigious institution, and to increase revenue. These needs, combined with a renewed interest by the academic center in solidifying referral networks, generated the climate for a new effort in cancer care delivery. The first three goals of the RCOP were to:

1. Bring state-of-the-art cancer treatment and prevention to [multiple sites in] rural Virginia.
2. Train rural community physicians and nurses to manage cancer pain, complications, and emergencies in the absence of the RCOP team.
3. Keep patients with cancer in their own community for diagnosis and treatment whenever possible.

Other goals included bringing clinical trials to the community and evaluating the cost-effectiveness of the program. The program was designed to support the rural hospital; all care including chemotherapy was and is given in the hospital. Part of the reason was coverage and billing, part was to keep the hospital whole. Another quote from the paper:

The oncologist-primary physician interactions are critical to safe and effective care of rural patients with cancer. Primary doctors seemed particularly satisfied that the same two oncologists attended each clinic. The RCOP team adopted an approach to community physician education and practice modification based on management theory about change in organizations [by Eisenberg]. These principles include creating an educational need, becoming opinion leaders, enlisting local physician leaders as agents of change, and following up with curbside discussions. For example, because the safe care of neutropenic patients was critical to the success of the program, the first RCOP tumor board addressed this topic. Rural internists, interested in the care of patients with cancer and supporters of the program, reviewed the practical aspects of neutropenic management and were enlisted to pass this information on to other primary physicians. As a result [of these and other efforts], changes in prescribing pain medication and referral of patients for clinical trials and better utilization of the academic center [also] have been observed.

Medical oncologists from Richmond and radiation oncologists from VCU visit to see patients on a regular basis (3-4 times a month in this case), and provide phone consultation as needed. For special needs or tests, a VCU van is available to transport patients to Richmond and back. Radiation facilities have been developed nearby in recent years so travel of patients to Richmond has become relatively rare.

The success of the RCOP has been documented in the large number of patients cared for locally, the earlier referral of patients suspected of having cancer, and the financial neutrality or gain from the program for the sponsoring hospitals. Examples : the number of patients receiving chemotherapy locally rose from zero to 100%. Breast-conserving surgery rose from 20% to 70%. Breast cancer that was Stage 1 or 2 at diagnosis rose from 59% to 79%. Oral and intravenous morphine use for cancer pain was zero; after the RCOP was established, prescriptions increased dramatically.

The program has been recognized in several ways: it received line item support from the Commonwealth of Virginia; it received the national Jesse Ball DuPont Award; it was featured on a Public Broadcasting Service television special on rural medicine; and it has received additional funding from the Commonwealth of Virginia, religious groups, and private donors to enable the continuation of its work. (Patient care dollars could never cover the cost of travel and time.)

RCOP is not the first or only cancer outreach program located in a rural community. Similar programs have been active in Vermont, South Carolina, Hawaii, and Washington State; some have been organized by private oncology practices.

The site that Desch described in the opening quote of this essay is one at which he has been the visiting oncologist from the start to the present day, even though he left VCU for private practice at the Virginia Cancer Institute (VCI) 7 years ago. His practice supports this effort to some degree. Despite the fact that there are no chemotherapy or laboratory revenue offsets, and no state support for private practice doctors similar to the support for academic doctors at VCU, Desch and his partners at VCI think this is a worthwhile effort, though it would be more profitable to see patients in Richmond. His 17-year relationship with the community at Rappahannock General Hospital in Kilmarnock, Virginia, has played a key role in its development. But as any oncologist knows in his or her bones, any successful program has terrific nurses behind it. In this case it is Ms Connie Deagle and her staff.

The "oncologists that make me proud to be one" described above are mostly not trained oncologists, but include nurses and primary care doctors; anyone who cares for patients with cancer. In this sense an "oncologist" includes anyone who cares enough about there patients to learn about them personally and about their diseases, and invests time, energy and emotion in their care. In my mind, some parents of my childhood leukemia patients were sufficiently knowledgeable and engaged in their child's care to be "oncologists." And in my years at St. Jude, we had a geographically widespread cadre of pediatricians and internists who gave chemotherapy, provided by us, to patients in their offices. We trained and supported them, we had annual seminars for them to bring them up to date, they liked being involved and the families appreciated not having to travel to Memphis so often.

What the efforts of the staff at VCU, the oncologists at VCI, and their local partners teach us is that determined leadership at both ends can improve the care of underserved patients with cancer. And it shows us that the care of rural patients with cancer can be as good as one can receive anywhere, and that it can be delivered with warmth and concern in a familiar environment by members of the patients' own community, a key determinant of the quality of life for many patients.

25 December 2005

"Concierge Medicine" and Other Trends

RECENTLY, I HAD AN ANNUAL CHECK-UP by my personal internist. He and his office staff were thorough, efficient, and friendly as usual, but at the end of our medical discussion he said he wanted to notify me that he was changing his practice. After "hyperventilating over this" for months, he decided he would convert it to a "concierge practice." He said his partners had already made the change and he now would follow.

He said he and his partners felt they no longer could practice the kind of medicine they desired under current conditions. They had taken on more patients and had spent less and less time per patient in the face of declining reimbursement in order to pay the bills. He also didn't like the idea of handing off the after-hours calls to "someone you don't know." He said he had 2,500 patients in his personal practice and he found himself rushing through visits just to finish. They had hired two new physicians in the past year but had to let them go because they didn't want to work the same schedule as he did.

He described his new "concierge practice" as follows. He (via a company that arranges these changeovers, MDVIP) would notify all his patients of this pending change and invite them to an explanatory presentation. The gist of the new practice is that he will have only 600 patients who are each willing to pay him an upfront fee of $1,500 per year, in addition to his regular fees. He will not pre-select the patients; they will be the first 600 who sign up. In this model, he will schedule more time for each patient, spend more time on prevention, health promotion, and counseling, become more involved in overseeing care given by sub-specialists and will "always" be available by phone or pager.

My wife and I both are under his care and when I brought the news home, her reaction was instantaneous—"He is an excellent doctor, takes good care of me, keeps me well informed, and I trust him. We fully discuss suggested treatments and he always values my preferences. Also, I don't want to start all over with a new internist. I will be the first to sign up." Although I agreed completely with her assessment of his talents, my response was more measured. I trust him, but something about this didn't sit quite right and I wasn't sure what it was. So I did some thinking.

I was curious about the finances. First, only people able to pay the annual $1,500 fee could sign up. Second, his practice is in a relatively affluent area, so it was a safe bet on his part that he would get his 600 patients. Third, $1,500 times 600 equals $900,000. Let's say the transition company takes 30% of the upfront fee (I am guessing), that leaves $600,000. Overhead costs of 60% would leave $240,000 in personal income *before* the collection of ordinary fees. In addition, reducing the practice by 75% would certainly lead to a similar reduction in staff and other overhead costs (the whole practice would be reduced to 1,800 patients from 7,500). Fourth, I don't know what my internist's personal income has been, but a 2005 survey of the annual personal income of busy, mid-career general internists in my area is a median of $176,000 and a 75%ile of $210,000 after overhead expenses. I can't say what a "fair" income is for any particular physician and I have no data on other factors that may influence his actual bottom line.

I do believe my doctor made this change for the right reason: so he can deliver better, more satisfying care at a more personal and less hectic pace. And like it or not, we live in a strongly capitalist society with all its strengths and weaknesses. Economists would say that as long as the playing field is level, the buyers (my wife and I in this case) have reasonable alternative options, and there is no monopoly, there should be no complaint, at least from a business point of view. And concierge medicine is indeed big business (see www.MDVIP.com). For an annual fee MDVIP and other companies manage the transition and market the concept. With a whole new source of financing uncovered, can Wall Street be far behind?

Then I stepped back and tried to depersonalize the issue. I realized that my little episode is taking place in the much larger arena of American medicine, which is facing seismic forces that have been developing for some time. Here is a sample of these trends that I believe are linked to one another, and to my episode.

Doctors

More recent medical graduates don't want to work the long hours that once was the rule. They want a different lifestyle with more leisure and family time, less night call, less hospital rounding. Furthermore, fewer and fewer medical graduates are going into primary care practice. A study published in *Academic Medicine* reported that in 2003 only 27% of residents had chosen careers in primary medicine and only 19% of medical school juniors said they would become primary care doctors; both numbers are much lower than in the past.[1]

Patients

Patients are being asked to take greater and greater responsibility for their care. Some of this is good, too much is not. It has been a mantra of patients and advocacy groups that patients need more information; doctors, pharmaceutical companies, and the internet have responded with a tsunami of information. The problem is that patients not trained in medicine (or even if they are) may have a very difficult time sifting out the chaff or even choosing from among the often confusing "good" choices. Referral to sub-specialists (which patients often demand or seek out independently) is far more common today, after which the primary care doctor may become disconnected from his patient. It is often up to the patient to maintain contact with the internist. This trend has, in many cases, put more distance between doctor and patient.

A 2005 front-page article in *The New York Times* describes this dilemma in graphic detail.[2] With case studies it points out that patients want more say in their management, but the handoff of decisions from doctor to patient may be clumsy and second opinions may simply confuse matters and put even more pressure on the patient. As the author, Jan Hoffman, explained when a patient insisted on staying with her doctor despite less than ideal results for her difficult problem, "It is impossible to overestimate the bracing impact of that old-fashioned guide, the doctor who can be a patient's constant, her polestar."

This shift of responsibility is engrained and growing. Patients test their own blood sugar and take their own blood pressure, and many make difficult decisions without confident advice from their doctor, without an "old-fashioned guide." Some blame the risk of litigation for this shift; I think that is a very small part of larger social changes, especially patients morphing into consumers, the changing lifestyle and professional expectations of practicing physicians, and the declining reimbursement for cognitive and psychological services compared with technical procedures.

Finances

Although most physicians do quite well financially, the rising cost of health care and the reaction of payers and employers have gradually squeezed their incomes–primary care doctors the most. They have no lucrative technical services to offer or chemotherapy to resell, so they are almost totally dependent for income on the traditional services of examination, assessment, and management. From many payers, and especially Medicare and Medicaid, that payment is totally inadequate for the time, angst, and intellectual and emotional capital required to do the job well. This has caused physicians to see more patients to maintain staff and income. Also, today's Byzantine billing systems require a large staff to manage the paperwork and cause endless frustration in today's practices. And, frankly, most doctors are poor businessmen (maybe "disinterested" is a better term), so they are attracted to simplified models like concierge medicine.

Thus far, concierge medicine has been limited mainly to primary care medicine. But there are other examples that have long operated on the same principle of an upfront premium cash payment from patients: cosmetic surgery; VIP suites in famous medical centers; and in some cases, bone marrow and organ transplantation. The potential scale of the current movement is, however, far greater because the per capita entry fee is within the reach of many more people.

After this long rumination, I am left with few answers and many questions. Who will take care of the 1,900 patients my doctor will no longer care for? And the other 3,800 patients his partners have already shed? Was my doctor's "hyperventilating" and apologetic demeanor an indication that he sensed that something wasn't right about it? Were his hesitancy and my own unease arising from the same place? Was it something in our medical training or the quiet nagging of the idealism most of us still have? Is this just another adaptation of medical practice, as from horse and buggy to automobile, or office microscope to an efficient and cost-effective for-profit lab? Or is concierge medicine another sign of the increasing industrialization of medical care, the patient becoming like just another consumer buying a car? And if so, is that also a sign of the erosion of a proud and noble professional ethic?

I don't know, but I do worry about it.

25 September 2005

References

[1] Garibaldi RA, Popkave C, Bylsma W: Career plans for trainees in internal medicine residency programs. *Acad Med* 80:507-512, 2005

[2] Hoffman J: Awash in information, patients face a lonely, uncertain road. *The New York Times*, August 14, 2005

BEING A DOCTOR

Concierge Medicine Revisited

I AM REVISITING THE DECISION of my personal internist to change his practice to the concierge medicine model. His two partners had previously made the switch and, after "hyperventilating over this" for months, he decided to join them (*see pp 114-117*). Although I agreed completely with my wife's assessment of our internist's talents, my response was more measured. I trust him, but something about this didn't sit quite right and I wasn't sure what it was. I calculated the income and concluded that he likely would be substantially better off.

So to summarize the advantages he described for his practice: fewer patients; greater accessibility of patients to him; more time for each patient; more time for prevention and other non-reimbursable services; more time for his personal life. He also viewed these advantages for the patients in his new practice, i.e. greater accessibility (24/7 by phone or pager), more time per visit, and more engagement with patients' sub-specialists.

I believed at the time that my doctor made this change for the right reason: so he can deliver better, more satisfying care at a more personal and less hectic pace. And I admitted that like it or not, we live in a strongly capitalist society with all its strengths and weaknesses. Economists would say that as long as the playing field is level, the buyers (my wife and I in this case) have reasonable alternative options, and there is no monopoly, there should be no complaint, at least from a business point of view.

To get a sense of how it has gone, I interviewed two patients participating in our internist's new system: my wife and myself. First I will point out that neither of us had any illness serious enough to require hospitalization, but both of us had been referred to sub-specialists for assessment and advice. In short, we are both in general good health and active both physically and socially. And second, we had been quite satisfied with our care before the change.

I asked my wife, Pat, what changes she has observed since the switch of our internist to concierge medicine. She said she doesn't believe there has been any change in the quality of her care; it was good both before and after the switch to concierge medicine.

However, she said our doctor has spent more time on and broadened discussions of prevention, weight management, and the like. She said the depth of their relationship is greater; he knows her better and doesn't need to rely only on the written chart. She said the response time to a phone call has been shorter by hours (it had never been days) and she has no wait at the time of an office appointment (waits had not been excessively long before).

But she made clear that she made the decision to stay with our internist because of him, not the new system. She had always had an open relationship with frank discussion and good dialogue so she could express her views and be sure they were taken seriously. That is why she stayed with him; she followed the doctor, not the promises made by the new practice structure. I asked her if it was worth the extra money. She said, "definitely, and I wish this was more [broadly] available in an affordable manner."

My own experience has been about the same as my wife's. The care is solid, as before, and accessibility is somewhat better, but I never thought it was objectionable before. In the beginning of the new model, I think our internist was trying a little too hard to behave in a manner that "justified" the extra payment, e.g., discussions in his office instead of the examining room or opening discussions about rare or insignificant issues. But he seems to have settled into a more natural pattern. The most important difference I have noticed is his more aggressive involvement with any sub-specialists we are referred to.

We were briefly discussing his new practice model recently when he volunteered that he personally is not making any more money than he did before (I did not feel it proper to ask for more details). However, he likes the new, more deliberate pace of his practice and feels he is doing a better job. And his private time has been enhanced. It seems that whatever hesitancy he had in changing his practice has evaporated.

I think my wife had it right. We stayed with our internist because of him, not promises touted by the practice model. The quality of care and level of trust were there before and after; the advantages of the new model would not alone have been substantial enough for us to change. This reaffirms for me once again of the primacy of the doctor-patient relationship in the practice of medicine.

10 December 2006

Doc-in-a-Drugstore?

RECENTLY IN THE *ATLANTA JOURNAL-CONSTITUTION* there was a full-page ad that got my attention and made me ponder the future of medicine once again. The ad was entitled, "Ultrasound Tests of Heart and Arteries." The first part of the ad offered a "Heart Attack Prevention Package." This consisted of three tests: an echocardiogram ultrasound test that "may detect enlargement of the heart, valve abnormalities, blood clots and tumors"; an electrocardiogram; and a "Hardening of the Arteries Test." All three tests cost $135 and are touted as "painless and non-invasive...and their combined cost is more than $1,300 at most hospitals."

The second part of the ad offered a "Stroke and Aneurysm Prevention Package," which also consists of three tests: a "stroke/carotid artery ultrasound test," an "abdominal aneurysm test," and a "blood circulation (arteriosclerosis) test." These tests also are painless and non-invasive. The price of these three is $95. And for a limited time, one can get all six tests plus a test for osteoporosis for a price of $179. The ad states that all tests are interpreted by board-certified physicians and the results with the films will be mailed directly to the person getting the tests. (Boy, that's an amazingly low price for all those tests; maybe they are being read in India.)

My initial reaction to the ad was, "tsk, tsk, what is this world coming to?" I saved the page and went back to it later and I must admit that my later response was more nuanced.

First, some facts: These tests will be offered initially at nine CVS pharmacies in the Atlanta Metro area by a company called Healthfair USA. At the website www.healthfairusa.com the company is described thus: "We are the next generation of preventive medicine. Featuring state-of-the-art, advanced mobile screening centers we call 'Health Coaches,' HealthFair USA provides vital, potentially lifesaving testing, including exclusive Advanced Biometrics. All this with unprecedented Joint Commission on Accreditation of Health Care Organizations (JCAHO) accreditation." Essentially, they have the equipment in buses that move to different locations based on scheduled testing.

Healthfair USA also offers corporate screening, which includes additional tests like cholesterol, blood pressure, and weight as well as a health risk assessment, advanced biometric testing, and active medical intervention. In the latter, a nurse will call and recommend referral to a disease management organization. I am certain that this is, or will be, a nationwide effort. I am guessing that CVS benefits from the traffic to their stores and/or through some financial arrangement for the use of its name and store sites.

Several issues occurred to me. I wonder what the clients are going to do with the films and the information. If one or more of the tests show definite pathology, I (and Healthfair USA) assume that the client will take the films and information to a physician who will provide appropriate follow up. Depending on the reader of the images, however, a substantial proportion of test results could have an equivocal interpretation. Either the client would go to a physician for clarification and follow-up or ignore the result. The client would become responsible for his or her own health care to a much greater degree than usual, something patient advocates and many patients want today. Without knowing the track record of the technicians and those reading the tests, it is impossible to speculate on the quality of the testing. The JCAHO accreditation provides only a modicum of security.

Here are some nuances. I have not made up my mind on the advisability of this approach to "prevention" ("early detection" might be a better description). Cardiovascular disease is not my field and the value of this service depends on factors that include the statistical probability of detection, the health risk and cost of unnecessary follow up testing, and the precision of both the diagnostic procedure and the analysis of the images. The initial expense is modest enough to be within the reach of many people, though the cost of follow-up could be substantial. The immediate physical risk is probably vanishingly small. Certainly other similar screening tests have been offered for years, e.g., total-body CT scans, and the public is accustomed to the idea of screening healthy people with mammography, colonoscopy, and determination of prostate-specific antigen and cholesterol levels.

So why am I uncomfortable with this particular approach to "prevention?" For one thing, it sounds too much like shopping at a supermarket without a shopping list; there is a high risk of impulse buying and buying things not needed or not even good for me. It also may mean not buying what I really need. In contrast, a patient's primary care doctor knows his or her lifestyle, medical history, and family history. Tests are ordered in this context and when screening tests are done, they would be appropriate for the medical history, age, and historical circumstances of the patient. The results of abnormal or suspicious tests would be explained and a proper referral made as needed. This seems to me both a more rational and a more complete approach.

But at heart, I think my uneasiness has little to do with these diagnostic tests; many diagnostics are, and probably should be, commodities—blood counts and chemistries come to mind. It has more to do with a persistent trend of the past several decades—the movement toward making a commodity of not just some tests, but *professional medical care*.

This trend began, in my view, in the early 1960s when Joseph Califano was head of the U.S. Department of Health, Education and Welfare (now Health and Human Services). If we think of medical policy of that era at all, we are likely to think of the Medicare Act of 1965. But Califano started another program that also had a lasting impact. He believed at the time that a major reason for the high cost of medical care was high physician fees and that the high fees were due to insufficient competition. His solution? Graduate more doctors to increase competition so that market forces would drive down the fees. He started a program of capitation and expansion of medical schools: the government paid medical schools a substantial fee for each new student slot in their classes and it subsidized the establishment of new medical schools and branches of existing schools, particularly state-operated schools.

Putting aside the issues of maintaining the quality of education and the downstream costs of this approach, this experiment of treating medical care as a normal capital market failed miserably to reduce the cost of care. As the number of physicians climbed, so did the number of specialists and the amount of expensive new technology. This continuing rise in the cost of medical care was powered (at least until recently) by the increasingly large pool of money available for medical care from both Medicare and employer-subsidized health insurance. This has been followed by the growth of other capital market features, such as direct-to-patient advertising by physicians and pharmaceutical companies, for-profit hospitals, and "managed care."

But medical care does not respond to market forces like an ordinary business, as we and our patients instinctively understand. So they and we are suspended between and influenced by market forces, affordability, access, litigation, increasing sub-specialization, physician and patient lifestyle changes, doctor shopping, unreasonable expectations, patient empowerment, and a tsunami of information in the media and on the internet.

It should come as no surprise that I don't have a solution for these issues. What I guess I am hoping is that we as physicians never lose sight of the wonder, privilege and responsibility of providing medical care. I am hoping that in this sea of money, hype and all the other forces that can move us to the dark side of our profession, that we keep our bearings and resist the movement toward commoditizing the medical care that each of us provides.

I would like to hear from many of you about your experiences and opinions regarding these issues so that we may better inform all of our readers.

10 July 2006

BEING A DOCTOR

A Doctor's Values from His Father

I HAVE BEEN CURIOUS FOR SOME TIME on the meaning of the pictures we hang on the walls of our offices. Photos of the wife and kids, diplomas and medical licenses are common clichés. Some hang art prints, photos of mentors and colleagues, or landscapes. The hangings may be influenced by who will enter the office besides oneself and intended to impress visitors (or oneself) of one's importance-with a medical board certificate, a plaque representing an award, or a photo with some dignitary.

I have hung all of these on my office walls at one time or another, but for the last 20 years a dominant theme has emerged. Except for two large photos of the mountains and pictures of two great artists, Willie Nelson and Pablo Picasso, the walls of my office (now in my home-no visitors) hold photos mostly of people who are my heroes. The eclectic mix includes Abraham Lincoln, Cesar Chavez, Donald Pinkel, the first director of St. Jude Children's Research Hospital, and one photo showing Giovanni Falcone and Paolo Borsellino. The latter were Sicilian prosecutors who started a major and successful legal attack on Mafiosi in Sicily, knowingly risking their lives; each was eventually killed by the gangsters.

Only one person, my father, is in more than one picture. One shows him behind of the counter of a diner (stools only, no tables), circa 1947, where he was a short-order cook. My father died in 1968, but he remains deeply embedded in my thoughts, values and prayers. In recent years on two public occasions at which I was honored, I have chosen to honor my father with a brief elegy. This was an attempt to convey how profoundly he influenced my values and, consequently, the choices I have made and opportunities I have had throughout my life. So here I honor him once more by repeating that short homage to him, perhaps reminding the reader of a father that also influenced his or her values.

The occasion in 1999 was my receiving the Stritch Medal from my alma mater, the Stritch School of Medicine of Loyola University. After recognizing the dignitaries and my family who were present, I talked about my father as follows:

I would like to tell you about the one person most responsible for my being here tonight. My father arrived in the United States from Italy in 1921 with the proverbial destination tag attached to his coat. He was 17 years old, all alone, an orphan, without education, speaking no English, and with only a few dollars. After a 3-week voyage in steerage on a steamer, he rode the train for 3 days from Boston to Fort Dodge, Iowa, where his older brother had been recruited years before to work in the gypsum mines for 2 years in exchange for steamer passage and citizenship. By then, his brother operated a diner where my father washed dishes.

After a few years he struck out on his own and went to Minneapolis where he found it difficult to find work with his limited English and dark complexion in a blond world. For a time there my father was homeless, and he developed a lifelong affection for the Salvation Army for taking him in. He eventually settled in Chicago and worked as a taxicab driver for many years. One day his barber, himself an immigrant from Sicily who did not drive, asked if my dad would take him in his taxi to the train station where the barber's wife and two children were arriving from the old country. The barber's daughter was a pretty 17-year-old who my dad fell in love with. A few years later, in the middle of the Great Depression, they were married and I was born 9 months and 11 days later—(close call Mom!).

My father was a wonderful man. He never had much materially. He never owned a home or a new car. He worked as a truck-driver and short-order cook and struggled as a financially unsuccessful small businessman. He didn't trust material things because they were evanescent and often brought more sorrow than joy. He believed in hard work and had enormous respect for education, deeply impressing both values on me. "Get an education; no one can take that away from you."

My father took joy in the little things of everyday life. He was a good cook and he thoroughly enjoyed a good meal, a cup of black coffee with 3 spoons of sugar and one spoon of bourbon, or the first fresh figs of the season. Every October he loved to make wine in the basement where he was the brains and I was the muscle.

My father was curious, open-minded, and he liked to try new things, an example that proved instrumental for me in my life and career. Most important, he was a kind and gentle man who genuinely liked people in all their diversity. He rarely spoke ill of anyone and never gossiped maliciously. He forgave easily and quickly. And he loved his family above all.

It is to his values that I have always aspired, never quite matching him. He was a better man than I am. Despite his rapidly failing health, he encouraged me to take the job at St. Jude in Memphis in 1967, leaving him and Chicago for the first time. Eight months later, shortly after his 64th birthday, about my age today, my father died–and after 31 years I still miss him.

So you can see that without his example, his values, and his encouragement, I wouldn't be here. This Medal belongs to you Pop.

10 June 2005

BEING A DOCTOR

Making an Oncologist – the Chicago Cubs Factor

WHAT INFLUENCES US TO CHOOSE the specialty of oncology has always interested me. Today there are many training programs and role models for medical students and house officers to emulate. But when I completed my internal medicine residency in 1963 and started a fellowship in pediatric hematology (that's another story), there were few formal training programs in oncology; the American Society of Clinical Oncology did not exist; there were no subspecialty board certifications for hematology, medical oncology, or pediatric hematology-oncology. At that time, there were many locations where only radiation oncologists and surgeons gave chemotherapy.

The relatively few full-time medical oncologists often arrived at their professions via other medical activities. The migration from hematology was the most common, but others came from a variety of specialties and activities as diverse as endocrinology (studies of hormone-dependent cancers) and from World War II studies of toxic compounds like mustard gas. As with physicians today, the choice of subspecialty in the early 1960s was influenced by a mentor, a patient, a family member, personal traits, or by unique or serendipitous circumstance. In my own case, the example and mentoring of Dr. Donald Pinkel, the first director of St. Jude Children's Research Hospital, made me a committed oncologist, scientifically as well as clinically.

Choosing medical or pediatric oncology was unusual and no easy matter in those days: medical and pediatric oncology were viewed with condescension by the pooh-bahs of academic medicine because they were "unscientific;" medical and pediatric oncology were mostly poor sister add-ons to hematology in medical schools (they thrived mainly at cancer institutes); the foundation of clinical trials was being laid with fits and starts; diagnostics for most cancer was primitive by today's standards; disfiguring and debasing gonzo surgery, including "super-radical" mastectomies and the fabled "hemi-corpectomy," was common; and the prevalent radiation oncology equipment was the cobalt-60 machine.

But the most defining feature of that time was the treatment–it wasn't very good and the great majority of patients died relatively quickly. Because of the stress of dealing with so many dying children, it was not unusual for pediatric oncologists to change specialties; some of my own colleagues switched to radiology, dermatology, neonatology, and radiation oncology.

While the support of mentors, our personality type, and the other factors noted above often influence our career decisions, I believe that the picture is more complex. I would guess that each of us could easily recall distant and seemingly unrelated personal experiences that instilled in us "life lessons" that helped us navigate this challenging field. Such recollections are seen, of course, through the fog of passing years. So with selective hindsight and a bit of puckish reconstruction, I have listed in roughly chronological order some of the character-shaping lessons that I believe helped me to choose and stay the course in pediatric oncology for 42 years.

Family Culture. I paid tribute to my father's influence on my values in an earlier essay (*pp 123-124*). But in this context his example of a deep mistrust of material possessions and of living within or below one's means served me well and later provided me the option of choosing extended post-residency training and an academic career which, of course, I did. **The lesson:** Live below your means and keep your options open as long as possible.

High School Football. All the coaches were "old school" in the early 1950s. Pre-school summer practices were brutal: twice a day in full pads and uniform in the August heat and humidity with no drinking of water during practice (I did say old school), and punishing scrimmages to see who could "take it." We had snug-fitting leather helmets with no face masks; I think all they protected was our ears from being torn off while blocking. We all talked about quitting, but few did. I wasn't a very good player and I rarely started, but I played well enough and the experience was invaluable. **The lesson:** I was capable of persevering under severely trying circumstances (handy insight for an oncologist).

Holding Retractors. Like many medical students, my choice of specialty changed several times before I made my final decision. I loved surgery...in theory. But after hours of holding retractors and doing all the other related chores (not very well), I decided that surgery wasn't for me. I didn't see myself getting enough satisfaction out of the operating room to make up for the rest of it. **The lesson:** The manual and technical aspects of medicine did not suit me as well as the intellectual.

Homer. No, not the Greek poet. Homer was a 5-month-old African American baby under my care during the pediatric elective of my medicine residency. He was a beautiful, chubby, happy baby who was always glad to see me. He had pyloric stenosis that eventually was surgically fixed without incident. For reasons I can't explain, caring for Homer helped me realize how much I liked taking care of kids; I still think of him over 40 years later. **The lesson:** Patients had much to teach us about ourselves, including what direction to take in our medical development.

Serendipity. Three examples: I moonlighted to support myself during med school as a hospital lab technician; that stirred my interest in hematology, which ultimately led to a career in oncology. One of the best hematology fellowships happened to be only two blocks from my residency institution so I could go to an interview at no cost; it also happened to be in a pediatric department, which ultimately turned me into a pediatrician. A colleague looked at a "hematology" job at a place I had never heard of then, the 4-year-old St. Jude Children's Research Hospital in Memphis, and suggested that it might be a better fit for me; I subsequently spent 24 great years at St. Jude. Each of these serendipitous events had a profound impact on the course of my career. **The lesson:** Planning is important, but chance can play a major role in a career; one should keep an open mind and not plan too rigidly.

The Chicago Cubs. I learned to read newspapers for pleasure from the sports pages of the *Chicago Tribune*. The Chicago Cubs' games were broadcast all summer; there was no TV and the radio announcers' dramatic renderings of the play made me a passionate fan. I suffered many years of the Cubs' legendary futility–they last won a World Series in 1908 and last played in one in 1945, when I was a 10-year-old. And even after leaving Chicago, I cannot remain completely detached from their fortunes or switch allegiance to another club. Maybe it was because I was born a few blocks from Wrigley Field. Maybe, as someone once said, a sports allegiance passionately held at 8 years of age is ingrained for life, like it or not. In any case, being a Cub fan entails accepting many defeats while retaining unquenchable hope. **The lesson:** Being a fan of the Chicago Cubs was excellent preparation for a life in oncology.

In summary, we all can point to major influences that led us to become oncologists, but I believe there are many seemingly minor factors as well. These "minor" factors may in the long run have been at least as important as the "major" factors, if not more so...and certainly are more interesting.

25 July 2005

Walker Percy

I AM INTRIGUED BY PHYSICIANS who also create literature. Some are known for their novels and stories that draw heavily on medical knowledge and technology: Sir Arthur Conan Doyle, Robin Cook, and Michael Crichton come to mind. Others write nonfiction based almost wholly on their medical experiences: Sir William Osler, Oliver Sachs, and Richard Seltzer, among others.

A third group writes "nonmedical" literature that often delves deeply into characters and philosophical introspection: Anton Chekhov, Oliver Wendell Holmes, Somerset Maugham, William Carlos Williams, Walker Percy, and Robert Coles represent this category with plays, novels, poetry, and nonfiction.

Those who wrote more recently—Williams, Percy, and Coles—are the most challenging and rewarding for me and are my favorites. Although their writing certainly was informed by their medical background, each used a far richer palette to explore fundamental aspects of the human experience. I have written an essay about Williams in these pages (*see pp 133-136*) and will write about Coles in the future; this essay is about Walker Percy.

Walker Percy (1916-1990) was raised in the South and attended the University of North Carolina and Columbia University College of Physicians and Surgeons, receiving his MD in 1941. He was training in pathology when he contracted tuberculosis and endured a 3-year convalescence.

Those 3 years were instrumental in several major life decisions he would make subsequently. During that time he read widely, fiction and nonfiction, but especially the existentialists Kierkegaard, Sartre, and Camus; the theologian-philosophers Aquinas, Pascal, and Marcel; and the great Russians, Tolstoy and Dostoyevsky.

These readings provided a jumping-off point for his subsequent writing and, it is safe to say, radically changed the course of his life. He worked as a physician for awhile, but soon, and seemingly all at once, he made the momentous decisions to marry, to leave medicine for full-time writing, and to become Catholic.

"Moral Self-Examination"

Percy's basic subjects were the human condition in modern times, American secularism, and the search for meaning and fulfillment in our daily lives. This is partly expressed by his comments in an interview by Robert Coles as he tried to explain his thoughts: "Let me try this on you," he said. "We ought to stop, every once in a while, and ask ourselves who we think we are. I am not just talking 'existentialism' here; I think I'm talking about moral self-examination—as in exactly who do you think you are?! There are times when we get so full of ourselves [that] 'we've lost all modesty.' I recall a teacher of mine in elementary school; she'd catch us being very 'clever,' lording something we'd discovered over everyone we could lay our hands on, and she'd call us to her, and she'd say: 'Now there, Walker, you sure are smart, you're clever as can be; and you're making sure everyone in the world knows it—the trouble is, that's not so clever, and it's not nice, either, because you've lost all modesty.'"

Percy thought we are too sure of ourselves, in our ability to cure with science all human diseases, to solve (or medicate) all our problems, questions, and anxieties, to know all truth and to satisfy all our desires. This attitude is promoted by the tidal wave of advertising that washes over us every day, promising to scratch the itch of every wish and fancy, to make us successful, celebrated, attractive, and desirable. And, when those promises, even when fulfilled, prove empty, we continue an endless, largely commercial, search for the next and the next and the next painless solution or next door to happiness.

Percy saw modern man, inundated and narcotized by the flood of consumerism, often settling into an unreflective and self-centered comfort zone of his own beliefs with automatic assents and a reflexive immersion in political party, church, profession, celebrity gossip, favorite TV program or football team; an intellectual and spiritual couch potato. He called it the "modern malaise."

That this same view persists four decades later is shown in a *New York Times Magazine* article by A.O. Scott.[1] The article begins by describing a new novel, *Indecision*, by Benjamin Kunkel: "[The book] concerns a young man living in Manhattan and trying, as the title suggests, to figure out what to do with his life. In his author's affectionate estimation, this young man is 'kind of an idiot.' Perhaps he may also be an especially representative kind of idiot and a familiar one: an alienation from his own experience brought about by too much knowledge, too many easy, inconsequential choices, too much self consciousness. Bred in a culture consecrated to the entitled primacy of the individual, he discovered he lacks a self, a coherent identity, maybe a soul. He feels he could be anyone."

Instead of *Homo sapiens*, he is *Homo viator*—Man the Wanderer. Percy could have written this.

Percy, too, was a member of the species *Homo viator*. But for Percy, a better translation of the Latin would be Man the Seeker, because Percy, unlike the passive protagonist above, was always asking the hard metaphysical questions concerning our existence, our purpose in being here, our happiness.

Percy explored these issues mainly in fiction, for which he is best known. His first book, *The Moviegoer*, published in 1961, was largely ignored until it won the National Book Award the next year.

The protagonist, Binx Bolling, is fascinated with movies because they make a place seem more real in the images on the screen (echoed by today's TV "reality" shows). His moviegoing has become an almost religious ceremony and more "real" than his own life.

The poet, novelist, and critic Marion Montgomery believes that Percy explained himself through Binx when he was asked in an interview about his being a "Southern" or "Catholic" writer: "He used Binx Bolling of *The Moviegoer* to talk about his own identity," she wrote in an essay.

"His concern is at a level deeper than the American anthropological concern with 'religion' and 'race' and 'local history.' Binx is a figure of modern man as wanderer...a wanderer within a limited local compass: a small geography that provides all the complexity of place as one might discover the world over, insofar as man is a wayfarer, that is, insofar as man is a *soul seeking its cause as a 'self'* [emphasis mine]. What is missing [in Binx] is the recognition of the full sun upon reality, to be encountered only if one abandons the tunnel vision of the self trapped in the cave of self-awareness, the Cartesian curse."

In other words, the increasingly individualistic modern man is very much alone (a tenet of existentialism). But with that individual freedom comes the awesome responsibility to find meaning. Some, especially existentialists, despair of finding any meaning. Many others search for meaning in a BMW or "six-pack abs" or cosmetics or "escape" to a tropical island.

Beyond Materialism & Modern Science

Percy believed that too few of us are willing to make that difficult journey toward the transcendent, that which is beyond materialism and modern science. Unlike that song of the 1960s, we rarely ask, with serious effort, "What's it all about, Alfie?"

This is heavy stuff. As described by Carl Olson, "While many novelists are content to be literary dermatologists, Percy was a literary surgeon—or better yet, a literary coroner—cutting beneath the skin and examining the very blood and guts of the modern man."

Olson quotes musings by Binx Bolling in *The Moviegoer* about what he is looking for. Bolling repeats a question asked of him and responds:

"What do you seek—God? You ask with a smile. I hesitate to answer, since all other

Americans have settled the matter for themselves and to give such an answer would amount to setting myself a goal which everyone else has reached—and therefore raising a question in which no one has the slightest interest. For, as everyone knows, the polls report that 98% of Americans believe in God and the remaining 2% are atheists and agnostics— which leaves not a single percentage point for a seeker. Have 98% of Americans already found what I seek or are they so sunk in everydayness that not even the possibility of a search has occurred to them?"

These themes and analyses in Percy's exploration are expanded in his subsequent books, like *Love in the Ruins* and *Lost in the Cosmos*.

"Huge Gap in Scientific View of World"

Finally, in other interviews and writings, Percy provides some explanation of the trajectory of his thought over time: "What did at last dawn on me as a medical student and intern, [and I as] a practitioner, I thought, of the scientific method, was that there was a huge gap in the scientific view of the world...science could not utter a single word [on] what it was like to be an individual being living in the United States in the Twentieth Century."

He believed that Science had extensive axioms and theories about the material world, but not about humans. But Percy was not anti-science and certainly not anti-intellectual. He made a distinction between science and "scientism," which my dictionary defines as the belief that science can explain everything. He said, "'Scientism' can only be considered an ideology, a kind of quasi religion—not as a valid method of investigating and theorizing which comprises science proper—a cast of mind all the more pervasive for not being recognized as such [and] one of the most potent forces which inform, almost automatically and unconsciously, the minds of most denizens of modern industrialized societies like the United States."

I read Percy not because I fully understand and accept everything he says. I read him because he explains compellingly that ours is an endless journey that too easily becomes stuck in a narrow, rotating gerbil cage going nowhere, in a habit of the routine acceptance of prevailing views, and of what other people—church, state, or science—maintain as truth and man's place in the world.

And, finally, I read Percy because he affirms the importance of a search for meaning, of transcendent values, of the "searching soul."

(I am indebted to the writings on Walker Percy by Marion Montgomery, Richard Purtill, Carl Olson, and Robert Coles for invaluable background information and quotations.)

25 October 2005

Reference
[1] Scott AO: Among the believers. *The New York Times Magazine*, September 11, 2005

BEING A DOCTOR

William Carlos Williams

I HAVE MET, WORKED WITH, OBSERVED, AND READ about hundreds of physicians in the 50+ years since I entered medical school. There are many who I have respected, usually for their medical skills, intellect, or efficiency. Some I have deeply admired, often for their humanity, their view of medicine as a calling and a sacred trust, or for the personal sacrifices they made for their patients and profession. And a handful has stimulated not only respect and admiration, but also a sense of awe and wonder. I would like to tell you about one of the latter, an American physician of my grandparents' generation who I never met, but have read about extensively.

William Carlos Williams was a general practitioner and pediatrician in Rutherford and Paterson, New Jersey. He cared for a working-class, mostly poor, immigrant population early in the last century, through the Great Depression of the 1930s, when house calls were a regular part of each day, and thereafter until his death in 1963. Why he is special, and the only reason I know of him, is that he was also a poet, probably the greatest successor to Walt Whitman as a uniquely American poet, one who used common language in an uncommon way. He wrote about ordinary people and everyday things in his community and his practice. It is fitting that his books follow Whitman's alphabetically on my bookshelf.

Dr. Williams, whose mother was from Puerto Rico, hence the middle name from her brother, was drawn to the arts at a young age and spent his life as a full-time physician while trying to be a full-time poet. So he wrote in his carriage while on house calls, between patients, and after office hours, "stealing" time from his practice and often complaining of overwork and the lack of time for writing. But despite the urgings of his colleagues in the arts, he refused to give up his practice to write and refused lucrative Manhattan practices.

Listen to Dr. Williams talk, first about "The Practice" from his autobiography.[1]

"It is the humdrum, day-in, day-out everyday work that is the real satisfaction of the practice of medicine; the million and a half patients a man has seen on his daily visits over a forty-year period of weekdays and Sundays that make up his life. I have never had a money practice; it would have been impossible for me. But the actual calling on people, at all times and under all conditions, the coming to grips with the intimate conditions of their lives, when they were being born, when they were dying, watching them die, watching them get well when they were ill, has always absorbed me. I lost myself in the very properties of their minds: for the moment at least I actually became *them*, whoever they should be, so that when I detached myself from them at the end of a half-hour of intense concentration over some illness that was affecting them, it was as though I were re-awakening from a sleep. For the moment I myself did not exist, nothing of myself affected me. As a consequence, I came back to myself, as from any other sleep, rested."

And more about his patients and society:

"I don't care a rap about what people are or believe. They come to me. I care for them and either they become my friends or they don't. That is their business. My business, aside from the mere physical diagnosis, is to make a different sort of diagnosis concerning them as individuals, quite apart from anything for which they seek my advice. That fascinates me. From the very beginning that fascinated me even more than I myself knew. For no matter where I might find myself, every sort of individual that is possible to imagine in some phase of his development, from the highest to the lowest, at some time exhibited himself to me. I am sure I have seen them all. And all have contributed to my pie. Let the successful carry of their blue ribbons; I have known the unsuccessful, far better persons than their lucky brothers."

And finally, he speaks about his poetry, for which he began to be recognized by literary critics only late in life.

"...I have never felt that medicine interfered with me but rather that it was my very food and drink, the very thing which made it possible for me to write. Was I not interested in man? There the thing was, right in front of me. I could touch it, smell it. It was myself, naked just as it was, without a lie telling itself to me in its own terms."

As with medicine, poetry was not a pastime for him, which was made clear in his ever-present red notebook:

If I did not have
        verse
I would have died
or been
a thief

So we hear a man deeply committed to his profession, his patients, his community, and to his poetry. The four are fused, inseparable, and interdependent, nourishing and revealing secrets to one another, about his patients, and about himself.

Dr. Williams wrote many poems, his magnum opus being the book-length "Paterson," in which he writes about the city, the times, and especially the people in all their glory and decadence, disease and health, joy and sorrow.[2] His style of writing is not ornate, but direct and tangible, though not necessarily simple or straightforward. In "A Sort of Song" he describes his style, using a metaphorical snake and flower; the parenthetical phrase in the second stanza is his famous line on poetry:

Let the snake wait under
his weed
and the writing
be of words, slow and quick, sharp
to strike, quiet to wait,
sleepless.

—through metaphor to reconcile
the people and the stones.
Compose. (No ideas
but in things) Invent!
Saxifrage is my flower that splits
the rocks.

He also wrote "The Doctor Stories" and poems about his practice and patients, some of which were compiled and introduced by Dr. Robert Coles, himself a famous physician and author.[3] As Dr. Coles says of them, "...the sheer daring of the literary effort soon enough comes to mind—the nerve he had to say what he says. These...accounts meant to register disappointment, frustration, confusion...or, of course, enchantment, excitement, pleasure...These are stories that tell of mistakes, of errors in judgment; and as well, of one modest breakthrough, then another—not in research efforts of major clinical projects, but in that most important of all situations, the would-be healer face-to-face with the sufferer who half desires, half dreads the stranger's medical help."

Needless to say, "The Doctor Stories," which I have read several times over the years (and that I highly recommend), were the final steps in elevating Dr. Williams to the upper level of my pantheon of doctors. He was by no means a saint and often a curmudgeon, but he worked hard every day at his passions, medicine and poetry. In both his practice and in his art he respected his poor, societally insignificant patients enough not only to care for them, but to listen to them, to study them, to understand them, and to write about them in all their humanity.

I am awestruck by his perseverance, sensitivity, artistic talent, and his commitment to the medical profession, which for him was clearly a calling and a sacred trust, as well as the lifeblood of his art. Though he died over 40 years ago, in his stories and poems he still has much to teach us about being a doctor, and about life.

10 October 2004

References

[1] Williams WC: *Autobiography of William Carlos Williams*. New York, NY. New Directions Paperback, 1967

[2] Williams WC: *Patterson*. New York, NY. New Directions Paperback, 1995

[3] Williams WC, compiled by Coles R: *The Doctor Stories*. New York, NY. New Directions Paperback, 1984

BEING A DOCTOR

Influential Books

LIKE MANY PHYSICIANS before and during their formal medical training, I was an avid reader of non-technical books about medicine, such as biography, essays, and fiction. A few of these books had a profound and lasting impact on my thinking and values so that even today, decades later, I have vivid memories of the issues, triumphs, and difficulties they addressed. My top three such books: *Microbe Hunters* by Paul de Kruif (initially published in 1926)[1]; *Arrowsmith* (1925) by Sinclair Lewis[2]; and *Aequanimitas* (1904) by Sir William Osler.[3]

Of course, the impact of books depends not only on the topic and skill of the author, but also the frame of mind of the reader at that specific time. All three fed my burning idealism, an unformed mixture of saving mankind, practicing medicine with utmost skill, and satisfying my scientific curiosity. These and other books helped move me gradually from seeing medicine as the fantasy depicted by Hollywood in the Dr. Kildare movies to seeing medicine as a vocation, a noble calling.

Microbe Hunters describes the work and the environment of scientists and physicians who explored, opened, and illuminated the world of microbiology.[1] Written for the general public with flair and suspense, a bit like the Western paperbacks of its day, it also has scientific heft and accuracy. I first read it as a teenager when my favorite sections were those describing the work of Pasteur, Robert Koch, and Paul Ehrlich; they still are my favorites. I was and am inspired by the struggles and perseverance of Pasteur and Koch who laid the foundations of microbiology and its application to curing human disease. Ehrlich strikes a special chord in me for his pioneering search for antibiotics and for essentially establishing the field of chemotherapy. This was dramatized effectively in the 1940 movie, *Dr. Ehrlich's Magic Bullet*, starring Edward G. Robinson.

Sinclair Lewis's *Arrowsmith* was dedicated thus: "To Dr. Paul H. De Kruif I am indebted not only for most of the bacteriological and medical material in this tale but equally for his help in planning the tale itself…"[2] I first read this novel during my pre-med years. It traces the career and struggles of Martin Arrowsmith, a physician-scientist in the fast-moving, fermenting world of microbiology in the early 20th century. The academic locale is based on the Rockefeller Institute (now Rockefeller University) in New York City, then a world leader in the study of micro-organisms and their diseases. I wanted to be Arrowsmith preventing and curing horrible diseases like plague, fighting the ignorance of peers and the wiles of academic politicians, risking my life to save lives, and tragically and heroically losing my devoted wife to the diseases we fought together in the tropics (the latter no longer seems attractive). It was an inspiring and, yes, heroic way of life.

I was in medical school when I first read *Aequinimitas* and was immediately captivated.[3] Here was a renowned physician, the first professor of medicine of the Johns Hopkins School of Medicine and one of the founders of the modern era of medicine, speaking directly to me about being a physician, a good physician. The book consists of a collection of Osler's addresses given over the years, many to incoming or graduating medical classes. They were inspiring and made me proud to be a budding member of the profession. But they also were practical, providing advice about how one should behave and what one should value. And most of all, his words rang true, refreshing and clarifying feelings and beliefs that were deeply, if vaguely, held.

The book was an immediate international hit. A section of Osler's preface to the 2nd edition describes the book's reception and intent, as well as his bedrock view of medicine as a calling akin to a religious vocation.

"I have to thank my friends, lay and medical, for their kind criticisms of the volume; but above all I have been deeply touched that many young men on both sides of the Atlantic should have written stating that the addresses have been helpful in forming their ideals. Loyalty to the best interests of the noblest of callings, and a profound belief in the gospel of the day's work are the texts...from which I have preached. I have enduring faith in the men who do the routine work of our profession. Hard though the conditions may be, approached in the right spirit—the spirit which has animated us from the days of Hippocrates—the practice of medicine affords scope for the exercise of the best faculties of mind and heart."

But Osler's head was not in the clouds. He continues, "That the yoke of the general practitioner is often galling cannot be denied, but he has not a monopoly of the worries and trials in the meeting and conquering of which he fights his life battle; and it is a source of inexpressible gratification to me to feel that I may perhaps have helped to make his yoke easier and his burden lighter."

The title address, Aequanimitas, was given to the medical graduates of the University of Pennsylvania on May 1st 1889, his last day at Penn before leaving for Johns Hopkins.

"...my tender mercy constrains me to consider but two of the score of elements which may make or mar your lives – which may contribute to your success or help you in the days of failure. In the first place, in the physician and surgeon no quality takes rank with imperturbability... [meaning] coolness and presence of mind under all circumstances, calmness amid storm, clearness of judgment in moments of great peril...It is the quality which is most appreciated by the laity though often misunderstood by them; and the physician who has the misfortune to be without it, who betrays indecision and worry, and who shows that he is flustered and flurried in ordinary emergencies, loses rapidly the confidence of his patients." He describes this quality in more detail and expresses regret that "some among you...may never be able to acquire it. Education, however, will do much; and with practice and experience the majority of you may expect to attain to a fair measure."

He goes on to describe the second and similar desirable element. "...the mental equivalent to this bodily endowment [imperturbability, is] a calm equanimity. How difficult to obtain, yet how necessary, in success and failure! One of the first essentials in securing a good-natured equanimity is not to expect too much from the people amongst whom you dwell." He continues that colleagues and patients are full of fads and eccentricities, whims and fancies and weaknesses, "which are not unlike our own."

Another passage also demonstrates the timelessness of his words despite the passing of a century. "I would warn you against the trials of the day soon to come to some of you –the day of large and successful practice. Engrossed late and soon in professional cares, getting and spending, you may so lay waste your powers that you may find, too late, with hearts given away, that there is no place in your habit-stricken souls for those gentler influences which make life worth living."

Among the 22 addresses are these titles, "Doctor and Nurse," "Teaching and Thinking," "Internal Medicine as a Vocation," "Nurse and Patient," "The Hospital as a College," and "Chauvinism in Medicine." In the latter, he lists the four great features of the profession of medicine -- its noble ancestry, remarkable solidarity, progressive character, and singular beneficence.

I will end this quick survey of Osler with several of his well-known quotes and biographical information. "One of the first duties of a physician is to educate the masses not to take medicine." "Look wise, say nothing, and grunt. Speech was given to conceal thought." "Live neither in the past nor in the future, but let each day's work absorb your entire energies, and satisfy your wildest ambitions."

A brief, but excellent biography of Osler can be found at www.whonamedit.com/doctor.cfm/1627.html. The site also has quotes, a list of his writings and a bibliography of literature written about him. The best major biography of Osler is the Pulitzer Prize-winning, *A Life of Sir William Osler*, by Dr. Harvey Cushing.

I believe there is no better inspiration and influence for medical students, residents and fellows than reading *Aequinimitas*. But reading Osler—and de Kruif and Lewis—still excites and inspires an old duffer like me as well.

10 July 2005

References

[1] De Kruif P: *Microbe Hunters*. New York, NY. Harcourt, Inc, 1996 (originally published 1926)

[2] Lewis S: *Arrowsmith*. New York, NY. Harcourt, Inc, 2002 (originally published 1925)

[3] Osler W: *Aequanimitas*. New York, NY. McGraw-Hill Professional, 3rd edition, 1932

BEING A DOCTOR

Protecting Patients from Us

DR. ROBERT WEBSTER AND I both joined St. Jude Children's Research Hospital right out of training at about the same time over 35 years ago. Rob is a PhD virologist who is internationally recognized for his laboratory and field work in influenza and severe acute respiratory syndrome (SARS), serving as an advisor to governments around the world, particularly in Asia.

But I know Rob best as a good friend and colleague. He had the most exotic career of any of us at St. Jude, traveling the world to obtain fecal and blood samples from ducks, chickens, and pigs, and culturing and typing the viruses, particularly influenza-type viruses. He studies the evolution of the viral immune phenotypes in an attempt to understand (and predict) the leap of such viruses from animals to humans. He would return from these excursions and give engrossing lectures that were scientific detective stories about of the genetic shifts in the viruses and which of them might be dangerous. He would remind us of the history of influenza epidemics and pandemics, like the deadly one of 1918 which killed far more American soldiers than the World War.

I had dinner with Rob recently and we talked about our families and what we were doing. When I told him I wrote a column he said he hoped I would write about a terrible problem that results in the unnecessary deaths of cancer and transplant patients and the elderly. The problem is the transmission of influenza virus from health care workers to patients, particularly those who are immuno-suppressed; they who are least able to fight the infection and, even worse, when infected continue to shed the virus, infecting others until they die.

He related several vignettes to make his point.

The Province of Ontario, Canada had such a bad outbreak of influenza in geriatric facilities from influenza passed from health care workers that they made a strict new policy. Any health care worker who fails to be immunized for influenza and contracts the disease is suspended from work without pay until they are no longer infectious. As a result the rate of infection of patients plummeted.

The SARS epidemic in Hong Kong was promulgated largely by health care workers from the index case, an ill physician from the mainland.

SARS is easier to contain than influenza. It is not as contagious and the patient does not begin to shed infectious virus until about the eighth day of illness, so quarantine is an effective means of control. Influenza is highly contagious and the virus is shed by the second or third day of illness, so quarantine is not usually an effective way to control spread.

Influenza, as we all know, may present as an apparently simple upper respiratory infection. I can recall Rob swabbing the throats of anyone at St. Jude who complained of a cold to look for the virus. We were a small place then and the basic scientists, physicians, nurses, and other staff ate together and crossed paths frequently during the day. We were often surprised when he told one of us we had influenza because we didn't feel very sick. (He also had a scientific reason for accosting us in the hallway, too; he wanted to know the phenotype of the viruses that appeared in Memphis as an epidemiological tool when connected with his worldwide network of colleagues.) This was a very important lesson to all of us: our apparent "winter cold" could kill our patients.

So what is Rob's advice to us who care for patients? First, get immunized. He feels strongly that all health care workers should be vaccinated because of the risk of passing the virus to so many vulnerable patients. A few days before writing this, we heard news that a major supplier of influenza vaccine had contaminated a large portion of its supply so there would be a shortage of vaccine. Rob believes that health care workers, particularly those who care for the elderly or the immuno-suppressed, should be given the vaccine preferentially in the face of the shortage.

What to do if one contracts influenza? Rob says there are two anti-virals that can be effective. Rimantidine, preferentially used in Canada, is relatively inexpensive, though resistance tends to develop rapidly, which makes it less successful for infected families. Tamiflu is one of the neuraminidase inhibitors. (Hemaglutinin and neuraminidase provide the two principle antigens of the viruses that determine their identities; for example, H5N1 is the strain of avian influenza now threatening Southeast Asia.) Tamiflu is more expensive than rimantidine but is effective, creates less resistance, and, if given early enough, can stop the spread of the virus.

So as a favor to my old friend, Rob Webster, and more importantly, as a favor to our cancer and transplant patients, get immunized and wash your hands often. And be especially alert that your upper respiratory infection this fall and winter could be due to influenza virus. Don't be guilty of negligent homicide.

25 October 2004

BEING A DOCTOR

Dealing with Change in Oncology

———⇒›●‹⇐———

I HAVE A LONG-STANDING INTEREST in how we physicians deal with change, especially changes in our working environment. In this essay I will eventually make a point about this relevant to the oncology environment. But before that, I will describe my observations of how many practicing physicians, community and academic, respond to change. All, some, or none of these observations may apply to you and your practice. At the very least, I am certain you will recognize others in these examples.

Facing change in our practices—caused or threatened by outside forces—is inevitable. When we are young and just starting out, we accept impending change more readily because we have little invested in the status quo and because we don't know any better. We accept change without a great deal of thought. This was brought home to me by observing my daughter and son-in-law. Both are physicians who completed their training in the early 1990s and entered a medical world consumed with the threat of managed care. But they seemed immune to the all the doomsday talk and hand-wringing. They had no history to compare to the proposed or actual changes and even if they were inclined to do so, no power to modify them. So they just motored on.

In mid-career, we are still somewhat connected to our training, do some clinical trials, and are more or less up to date. We still go to annual meetings and read articles in *Journal of Clinical Oncology* (JCO) or *Blood*. We accept change selectively and try to be proactive, if we have the time, but a growing practice and family consume almost all of our energy.

In the final third of our careers, we have become well-established professionally and domestically. We find it much harder to change in either sphere because there is much more at stake. We may not be up to date scientifically, but we usually know the latest indications for therapy. Whether the new medications are used appropriately depends on who is the judge. We may look at some of the abstracts in JCO, or maybe just the table of contents, or skip it altogether. Our experience is vast and our judgment excellent, we tell ourselves. Our patterns of care and referral conduits are entrenched. We have bought the second home in the Berkshires, the 32-foot sailboat, the BMW, or a new trophy wife. And if we weren't already, we probably became Red-Staters along the way. We have it pretty good, so we don't really want anything to change, least of all our practices, and will fight like hell to keep things as they are.

So all of us some of the time and some of us all of the time are relatively passive when facing changes in our practice environment. Either we let it happen and react, complain loudly but do nothing, or forcefully (and actively) resist any change. In all cases, the posture is essentially defensive. Our reaction to these outside forces rarely includes taking anticipatory action based on principle and/or offering viable alternatives.

Ironically, we often take anticipatory action with patients in our practices, as I will describe below. And there are those of us who, given the chance, will take the initiative regarding the practice itself, and I will give an example later.

Most of us do not use a passive approach to the practice medicine. We usually anticipate a change in our patient's condition, sometimes without solid evidence. We may ask them to return sooner, discuss the patient with a colleague or order some films or blood tests. We try to anticipate and get control of the situation before it deteriorates further. The contrast is revealing. We think ahead, adapt to shifting signs and symptoms, and intervene with dispatch when managing our patients. We are mostly passive, defensive, and reactive in managing our practice environment.

A case in point is our collective response, mainly through our membership associations, to the Medicare Modernization Act (MMA). You know the facts; here is a brief recap. The MMA was proposed by President Bush and passed by Congress mainly to offer a pharmaceutical benefit to seniors. Some viewed this as a cynical, purely political act to cement the vote of seniors and, by the way, to enrich pharmaceutical companies. However, others believed it would help needy patients. The two views are not mutually exclusive.

What was not fully appreciated at the time by physicians is that Medicare's pot of money is really two non-exchangeable pots: one for pharmaceuticals and one for everything else. Thus, the pharmaceutical benefit had to come from the pharmaceutical pot with no increase in the size of the pot. Congressional staffers had three main statistics to work with at that time: most of the ten costliest drugs for Medicare were prescribed by oncologists; an average of about 65% of oncology practice income came from the sale of drugs; and the average annual income of oncologists was $200,000 to $400,000, depending on geography and other variables. So we all know what happened: Congress moved to sharply reduce what Medicare could be charged for the oncology drugs. Average wholesale price went out and average sales price came in.

Our initial response, mainly through our professional societies and other organizations, was to cry foul and to paint a doomsday picture for our patients with cancer and for our practices. We rightly said that the reimbursement for seeing, examining, and advising a patient and family was ridiculously inadequate for the time spent with these frightened and depressed patients. We rightly said that the earnings from re-selling the drugs made up for the losses. Aggressive lobbying and other efforts were to no avail. We made what was largely an economic argument, ceding the ethical high ground of "providing drugs to those who cannot afford them" to Congress. Though some horse-trading was attempted late in the game, our reaction was mainly a call for a return to the status pro ante which, of course, failed.

Could this have been avoided? Maybe not, politics being what it is. But using my handy retrospectoscope, maybe if we had invested as much energy in improving reimbursement for managing the patient before the MMA was introduced, we might have been in a better position to withstand its impact. We justifiably could have made the case that the quality of care depends on many factors, but spending sufficient time with a patient is essential; the reimbursement system perversely places little value on such activities. But as long as the drug money was pouring in, there was little incentive to take such action, to take the high ground and push hard for fairly valuing time with the patient. Such an effort may not have succeeded, but it would have firmly established our position on the main issue at stake, namely, the quality of cancer care. Instead, Congressional staffers viewed us as "rich guys coming up here in Armani suits saying how poor they are" (an actual quote).

So why go over this old news? Because we have another opportunity to anticipate change, do the right thing, and take the high ethical ground. We face another intersection of economics and the quality of cancer care that can profoundly influence the environment of our practices. It is called "Pay for Performance" (P4P). Like many trendy phrases, P4P can mean many different things. To payers, it means controlling costs and gathering valuable data on the comparative performance of practitioners. To physicians, it may mean payers trying again to pick our pockets or pit us against our colleagues or burdening us with even more paperwork.

But I see it as an opportunity for us to influence the process and use it for improving the quality of cancer care while P4P is still in its infancy. We should take a stand that quality of care is the prime measure for any change. Cost matters, of course, but the danger is that cost, with its readily available numbers, will become the prime force. One approach is ASCO's Quality Oncology Practice Initiative (QOPI), which is growing and evolving. It provides a chance for oncologists to influence the shape and ethical ground rules of P4P. It is not yet clear how the economic issues of P4P will play out. But QOPI's focus is on the quality of cancer care, which can put the oncologist on the ethical high ground, whatever the direction of payers' efforts. An appropriate alignment of quality and reimbursement is a much more likely outcome if we anticipate and participate in efforts like QOPI.

10 Oct 2006

Retirement Adventures

MY FATHER WAS A "WORKING MAN." In his day (1904-1968), that meant he worked hard physically for hourly wages or for a meager income from a small business requiring 10-14 hours a day. In his generation, working men hoped to retire with a pension, which for the majority consisted only of Social Security. They eagerly looked forward to the day they no longer had to work. And although Social Security wasn't much, they could get along by living modestly as they were accustomed. But before reaching the traditional retirement age all too many became chronically ill and could no longer work or died; both happened to my father.

Times have changed. Though there are still many today just like my father, especially immigrants, the pay and benefits (until recently) have steadily improved for average working men. An even bigger change has been the increase in longevity. What do those men (and women) do with the 10, 15, or 20 more years after age 65?

My unscientific and unsystematic observation suggests that most of those retirees (or potential retirees) fall roughly into the following categories: 1) Do nothing in particular. 2) If finances allow, move to a nice climate, play golf, travel, and/or dive into one's hobby or other diversion. 3) Continue work out of financial necessity. 4) Continue work out of habit, to have something to do, to have a place to belong and sense of security, or for the continued enjoyment of the work. 5) Try new jobs to stay engaged and reinvigorated, e.g., volunteering, doing part- or full-time work using one's expertise, or starting a business. 6) Never retire, but continue doing the same work ad infinitum, or until retirement is imposed by illness or incompetence. My sense is that physicians and other professionals, just like today's salaried workers, would fall into one or more of the same categories depending on medical, family, and other issues.

But for me a more important and meaningful way to understand retirement and the likelihood of its being a happy time requires only two categories: active and passive.

Passive retirement would have included most working men of my father's generation. The opportunity to stop doing hard physical labor or working long hours was the goal. That is also true of men and women today who do hard physical labor. They often had no specific plans except to rest, putter around the house, to enjoy the grandchildren and the like. In other words, they would simply expand the time for things they already did and have time for "dolce far niente," a wonderful Italian phrase meaning "the sweetness of doing nothing." I have seen some professionals do this. Several older relatives chose this course, but most eventually had a major problem to deal with: boredom; more on that later.

Passive retirement also happens among professionals, who ordinarily do not do hard manual labor and who usually have the resources to do almost anything they wish. Many ease into retirement by doing less work and more leisure activity. Some, particularly in academic settings, "retire in place," that is, they pretend to be as active and productive as ever, but they are not, so they go to meetings, serve on committees, busy themselves with non-jobs, such as assistant vice dean for something or other, or just keep their head down and coast. They are boring, but never seem bored.

Active retirement can take on many forms. A good friend and colleague planned long before he retired to live in a warm place and play golf three or four times a week so he could improve his game and enjoy it more, and enjoy "*dolce far niente.*" His wife also golfed, so it was something they could do together. He was an eminent pathologist and turned down opportunities to work part time; he decided to cut the cord from his attachment to medical work. He has had a happy retirement with not an iota of regret. Other professionals plan to become avid travelers, take courses in Shakespeare, or begin planning to work at something different.

By definition, active retirement requires planning and preparation. Virtually every ad one sees on TV that deals with retirement addresses the financial aspects. This is not surprising since the ads are sponsored by insurance, investment, and annuity companies. But while financial planning is important, by the time one is seriously contemplating retirement, usually, the die is cast; it is difficult to substantially change one's financial position in 2 years and few take retirement seriously and do the necessary research, planning, and testing before then. So at that stage the financial planning is an exercise on what resources one has and how long they are likely to last.

As you can tell, I am an avid fan of active retirement. I think active retirement is an opportunity for adventure of one kind or another. The likelihood of boredom in passive retirement is high and can lead to excessive drinking and eating, depression, and becoming an unpleasant curmudgeon with no apparent joy in life. In my own case, the impetus for active retirement was powered by my aversion to boredom along with my compulsive need to plan ahead.

Five years ago this month, I gave up a perfectly good, well-paying academic job to try something different before I cashed in my chips. My father and both grandfathers died in their 60s so I had greater reason to retire then if I were ever going to try something different. Leaving familiar work, friends and colleagues, and financial security was not a step taken lightly, and I admit to harboring misgivings periodically. Planning resulted in my starting a one-man consulting business, which allowed me to stay intellectually engaged in cancer center activities. The work is part-time leaving time for unplanned activities such as volunteering at a local hospice, starting the Quality Oncology Practice Initiative at ASCO and writing this essay. I work from home so I have no commute, no employees or bosses, and much more time with my family. I thoroughly enjoy all these and other activities and none would have been possible had I not retired.

For most professionals, my advice is to plan an active retirement. You go around only once and you don't know how much time you have left, so don't wait too long.

10 August 2006

On Giving Advice and Offering Some

ADVICE COMES IN TWO GENERAL CATEGORIES. The first is bad advice, which includes useless, dangerous, or manipulative advice. Examples include "Take a bite out of this apple" and "Go (bleep) yourself." This category is the most important since correctly assessing the integrity and wisdom of the advice-giver allows one to put most advice in the trash, thus avoiding bad choices.

The other is good advice, that is, *potentially* useful advice from a trusted and insightful adviser. Even if one ultimately chooses not to take it, the viewpoint good advice provides helps one sort out the options. Good advice is not always welcome, of course, for example, advice to your daughter about whom she should marry.

There are two types of good advice. Practical advice usually deals with near-term decisions or actions. Examples include advice on how to deal with a difficult co-worker, advice from an experienced nurse on managing a patient, and where the best pizza is made, Chicago or anywhere else. Strategic advice usually deals with actions or choices that are likely to have a lasting impact, such as making a key career choice, developing a particularly useful or rewarding habit, or who your daughter ought to marry.

As one ages, the urge to give advice grows. There are several reasons for this. Since we are mortal, most of us have an instinct to leave something of lasting value that keeps our existence "alive," a kind of immortality. Also, seniors have probably given and taken enough advice, good and bad, to make them more discerning about what to pass on to others.

This is a sneaky way of leading up to my giving you advice. Using my own categories, I am far too modest to judge if my advice will be good or bad. (Now, really, would I give you bad advice?) But the advice will be coming from a ruggedly handsome fellow (that is what a Hollywood publicist calls an ugly actor), who is eminent and distinguished (that is how all professors think of themselves, whether they are or not), and has no conflict of interest in offering the advice (this one is mostly true, but more about that later).

The advice I offer can have long-lasting effects (mostly good, I hope) on the quality of your life and, perhaps, your career. It is aimed mainly at young people, young in age or in open-mindedness. (Full disclosure: this opinion comes from one who is approaching his 70th birthday.)

A point of information: I wrote a paper in 1999 that offered advice, "Understanding Academic Medical Centers – Simone's Maxims," which was directed mainly at younger people navigating a career in academia. I later enlarged and updated the paper and self-published it as a booklet entitled, "Institutions Don't Love You Back." An updated version of those maxims can be found at www.simoneconsulting.com.

Here is a list of my recommendations for a more fulfilling and enjoyable life. There are only two.

Keep a Journal

I received good strategic advice during my residency after I had decided to try for a career in academic medicine. (I can't remember the source...so much for giving advice being a ticket to immortality.) The advice was this: If you want to be an academic, you must learn to speak and write well; to do them well you must work at both. The advice continued that a good way to practice writing was to keep a journal. This, of course, is good advice for anyone, academic or not, who needs to communicate ideas and information to others.

So I purchased a bound notebook and began writing about family, work, books, movies, people, and places I had been. I wrote about decisions I was struggling with, religious faith, civil rights, dying patients, and anything else that interested or troubled me. I wrote any time I felt like it at no set intervals, with no regular format and no intention of writing a complete record of all my experiences; I also had no intention of writing for any audience or for publication, only for the practice.

In a matter of months, a strange thing happened. I was no longer writing to practice writing. I had developed the habit of writing as a means of conversing with myself, dissecting problems, letting off steam, mourning a loss, and describing a joyful experience. I wrote during night call, at my desk, on airplanes. I rarely re-read the entries because writing's main value was the act of expression.

I have been writing in my journal continuously for 45 years. There are 29 handwritten volumes with a total of over one million words, the equivalent of ten novels of 400 pages each. The journal became an important part of my life, helping me clarify my thinking, see through some of my foolishness, and achieve a modicum of wisdom. How many things in life can do that for you so easily and consistently for over four decades?

So my advice, regardless of your age, is that you buy a bound journal of 150 lined pages, light enough to stick in your briefcase, and start writing. For a month or so force yourself to write something, anything, at least once a week. If you do that, you likely will become hooked and have a lifetime friend, companion, mirror, and confidant.

Read Poetry

The next bit of advice is related to the first. After I had been writing in my journal for awhile, my writing had not improved. And then I found two suggestions from an article for beginning writers. First, get a copy of *The Elements of Style*, by Strunk and White. (E.B White was an editor and writer for the New Yorker and also wrote children's stories.) That short book with tips on writing more economically, effectively, and lucidly would become my writing conscience.

Second, to write well, it was important to read great books of literature so one may grow to know and sense what excellent writing looks and sounds like. The article specifically recommended reading poetry because a key feature of poetry that applies to all good writing is saying a lot in as few words as possible. And good writing means choosing exactly the right word and no more, an echo of Strunk and White.

At that time I had been reading some literature but not much poetry. So I began and found it difficult. Much of it seemed vague with unfamiliar word sequences and allusions. But I persevered and began to find the occasional poem that beautifully expressed a sentiment or observation. In time, I discovered two things: that I did not have to like all of it and that my taste and artistic sensibility, gradually refined, should be the arbiter of what I liked and didn't like. Over time I found that I liked authors who wrote in a variety of styles, from ancient Japanese and Chinese poetry, T.S. Eliot and William Carlos Williams, to contemporary poets such as Stanley Kunitz, Jane Hirshfield, Billy Collins, and Czeslaw Milosz.

Once again, the unexpected happened. My writing did improve, but I also became hooked on poetry and all the insights and intangible riches that it brings. Today about one-third of my personal library is poetry. Poetry at its best is subtle, suggestive, and at times mildly provocative. One must work at it a bit, as with any encounter with art, to get the most from reading it, but the dividends in pleasure and "seeing with new eyes" are more than worth it.

So here is my advice on how to start reading poetry. Write a check for $35 for a year's subscription to "Poetry," a thin monthly (published in Chicago, I might add) with a long and distinguished history. Put it on your bedside table and read a poem or two once or twice a week. Stick with it and I guarantee that you will find poems that you like (and don't like), your appreciation and discernment will grow with time, and soon you will be browsing the poetry sections at Barnes and Noble, Borders, or Amazon.com.

This advice is free and it comes from the heart.

25 August 2005

Chapter 5

MEDICAL ETHICS AND VALUES

Medicine is a profession that society has granted substantial independence of judgment and practice. How physicians respect or abuse this privilege is a passionate interest of mine. These essays describe actual and potential challenges to the dignity and nobility of medicine by individuals and organizations and my reaction to them. Money and power, as in all human endeavors, are often at the root of the problems.

Conflicts of Interest in Medical Practice

WHEN IN MY TRAVELS PEOPLE MENTION MY COLUMN[1] to me, they most often say they like the ethics essays best. I believe one reason is that conflicts of interest touch the medical conscience in particular because they erode not only the public's trust, but the physician's core values and personal view of him or herself as a dispassionate agent working first and foremost for the patient's good. Today's economic landscape of medicine presents a flood of opportunities for unethical material benefit. Most of us recognize and condemn obvious major conflicts, such as giving a drug that is much more expensive but no more effective or safe than a much cheaper alternative. More often it is the case that apparent or actual conflicts of interest are not only legal and commonplace, but we view them as quite innocent with a "no harm, no foul" attitude, like the donuts at tumor boards and the seminar dinners funded by drug representatives. We believe that we are not influenced to use the drug representative's hot new drug by eating the donut, so what's the problem and what ethical norm should we apply, if any?

As a result of the feedback from my columns, I have wrestled with these issues from time to time and most recently that process has taken me back to my childhood. When I was in public grade school I attended religious instruction classes at Our Lady of the Angels parish on Chicago's West Side. The classes were intended to prepare one for receiving the sacraments, such as Holy Communion and Confirmation, the latter at about age 12. The written instrument of instruction at that time was the Baltimore Catechism, a book that contained the basic tenets of Christianity in a question and answer format. I remember the appearance of the book vividly. It was about the size of a *Reader's Digest* magazine and had a soft silver-gray cover.

Today I remember few of the specific questions and the formulaic answers, but one of the admonitions for leading a holy life has remained vivid in my memory ever since and I believe that it has relevance to medical ethics. A word of caution: just because I can explain it to you doesn't mean I have always observed it in my life, but it is always there lurking in my conscience.

[1]*Simone's OncOpinion*, Oncology Times (*www.oncology-times.com*)

The admonition is to "avoid the occasion of sin," in other words, avoid putting oneself in a situation that provides the opportunity for sin. What stuck with me is that doing so was considered a sin in itself, even if the wrongdoing never actually happens. So inviting the possibility of sin is a sin. That seemed harsh and unacceptable to me as a preadolescent, but deep down I knew it was right.

Whether a sin is committed is a matter of conscience, of course, so a reliably accurate judgment of sinfulness by other human beings is impossible. Thus, when we establish ethical guidelines for our professional behavior in our secular lives, we develop standards that we human beings can judge. That is why we employ standards such as avoiding the appearance of wrongdoing as well as the actual wrongdoing. Some practical, secular examples follow.

Every time a college student goes to a fraternity party, he gets blind drunk. If we can agree that getting blind drunk is wrong, under this standard the act of his going to a frat party is wrong, even if this one time he doesn't get drunk.

When one is reviewing grants for the National Cancer Institute, one cannot review grants submitted from one's own institution, even if the investigator is unknown to the reviewer. Furthermore, one is usually asked to leave the room when that grant is being discussed. When serving on committees for the Institute of Medicine, one must publicly disclose financial or personal interests that might give the appearance of a conflict of interest, such as substantial stock holdings in a pharmaceutical company that might be at issue in the deliberations.

An example from journalism is the response Walter Mossberg, who reviews technology for *The Wall Street Journal*, gave to a query in his column of 28 April 2005.

Q: *I am wondering if you ever get paid by companies, in cash or kind, for any reviews or recommendations of their products that you make in your articles. I ask this because I have recently read that a number of reviewers in the media charge money for favorable opinions or mention of technology products.*

A: No, I don't. I neither seek, nor accept, money, or anything else of value, from the companies whose products I cover. I return any products I am lent for review, except for items of minor value which companies don't want back. In the case of these items, I either discard them or give them away in return for donations to charity.

I also don't accept trips, speaking fees or "editorial discounts" from companies whose products I cover. If I want a product I review for my own use, I buy it, at retail. And I don't own a single share of stock in any of the companies whose products I cover. Also, I never coordinate my reviews with our advertising sales department, and don't solicit or sell ads. On many occasions, I have written negative reviews of products from companies that advertise prominently in this newspaper, and positive reviews of companies that don't advertise.

While I can't speak for other reviewers at other publications, I believe that generally similar policies are followed by major reviewers in the best known print publications. It's unfortunate that a few so-called reviewers, mainly on television, do charge companies for mentions, and thus raise doubts in the public's mind about technology reviews in general.

Thus, the standard applied in the above examples is to avoid conflicts of interest, avoid the appearance of conflicts of interest, and publicly disclose any potential conflicts of interest.

The physician's relationship is different from the examples above in one major respect: it is a private relationship with essentially no outside oversight. Thus, the patient is dependent solely on the physician to act professionally and ethically. But since the patient has no way of knowing if that is the case and can look to no oversight body for assurance, the physician bears a much greater responsibility not only to avoid conflicts of interest, but also, insofar as possible, to avoid the appearance and the *opportunity* for conflicts of interest.

If one applied this standard to the practice of medicine, physicians would, for example, not sell drugs to patients at a profit beyond covering actual costs of purchase and administration, would have no pecuniary interest in a radiation therapy facility to which he referred patients, and would publicly disclose any potential conflicts of interest. In these cases, he would avoid the opportunity for a conflict of interest and would make transparent anything that might appear to be a conflict of interest.

But there are two confounding issues that complicate matters. First, what if one does not voluntarily put oneself in such a position, but is thrust into a sea of opportunity for recommending procedures or therapy based on their financial advantage? Human nature suggests that, unless diligently avoided, it will become easier and easier with time to convince oneself that all decisions are made ethically, or at least with a "no harm, no foul" approach, even if that were not the case.

Second, is it possible to practice oncology and make a living if one applied those standards? One might argue that the current reimbursement system conspires against such an approach. Some oncologists simply could not survive financially because of the grossly insufficient reimbursement provided for examining and managing the patient's care and for the long discussions with the patient and family that are commonplace on the practice of oncology. Doctors should be able to make a "living," whatever that means financially. The perversity of the current reimbursement system has been catalogued in detail by others. So what is one to do to both survive in practice and aspire to practice the highest standards of ethics? What is one to do to safeguard one's integrity under those circumstances? How do physicians in the trenches avoid conflicts of interest?

I don't have pat answers for these questions. But I am convinced that avoiding conflicts of interest is essential for sustaining the integrity of the practice of medicine. How one does so and what safeguards one puts in place to keep on that track will vary from practice to practice. I believe if one can be honest with oneself, satisfactory judgments can be made. Two signs of one's ethical success are an honestly clear conscience and no fear of our actions appearing on the front page of *The New York Times*.

25 May 2005

"The Stonemason" on the Integrity and Sanctity of Work

I RARELY READ WORKS OF LITERATURE COVER TO COVER a second time; the great majority I read through once and only portions thereafter. But a few I read cover to cover repeatedly, as if for nourishment or direction, assurance or inspiration. It is for these reasons that I re-read "The Stonemason," a play by Cormack McCarthy,[1] who is best known for his novels, such as *All the Pretty Horses* and *Suttree*.

The play is set in Louisville Kentucky in the 1970s and is narrated by Ben Telfair, a stonemason whose father, Big Ben, and his grandfather, Papaw, are also stonemasons (papaw is a common name for a grandfather in the South.) It is a masterfully written story of a family faced with the acute problem of Ben's wayward nephew, Soldier, who is in trouble with the law. The play has a number of important layers, but the soul of the work, and the reason I read it over and over, is Papaw, the 100-year-old stonemason. His passion intimately weaves the sanctity of work and craftsmanship into a single fabric with spiritual wisdom about what really matters in life. He reminds me of the craftsmen who built medieval cathedrals with pride of craftsmanship and with an acute sense of the nobility and sanctity of their work.

Ben recognizes the knowledge and wisdom that Papaw offers and he avidly tries to soak it up before Papaw is gone. When he realizes what a remarkable and unique resource his grandfather is, he says, "Oh I could hardly believe my good fortune. I swore then I would cleave to that old man like a bride." Neither Big Ben nor Soldier places a high value on Papaw's views of stonemasonry and his exacting standards.

During the course of the play, Papaw relates through Ben's narration what he knows and how he feels about stonemasonry, and not coincidentally, about life. He is also speaking to us about how one loves and respects his work: the truth of it, the wholeness of it, the essence of it. For Papaw, how he approaches his work is inextricably linked to how he views the world, how he treats others, and how this is all intertwined with his basic faith.

Here are excerpts from the play. While Ben and Papaw are working on a farmhouse, Ben the narrator speaks about stonemasonry:

"For true masonry is not held together by cement but by gravity. By the stuff of creation itself. The keystone that locks the arch is pressed in place by the thumb of God. When the weather is good we gather the stone ourselves out of the fields. What he likes best is what I like. To take the stone out of the ground and dress it and put it in place. We split the stone out along their seams. The chisels clink. The black earth smells good. He [Papaw] talks about stone in a different way from my father [Big Ben]. Always as a thing of consequence. As if the mason were a custodian of sorts. He speaks of sap in the stone. And fire. Of course he's right. You can smell it in the broken rock. He always watched my eyes to see if I understood. Or if I cared. I cared very much. I do now. According to the gospel of the true mason God has laid the stones in the earth for men to use and he has laid them in their bedding planes to show the mason how his work must go. A wall is made the same way the world is made."[1]

There are physicians who have the same respect, almost reverence, for their patients. Perhaps for them it is because the mystery of their lives is held together "by the stuff of creation itself" and deserves—no, demands—professional and personal respect.

Ben continues, describing the essence of the work. "So. It's not the mortar that holds the work together. What holds the stone trues the wall as well and I've seen him check his fourfoot wooden level with a plumb bob and then break the level over the wall and call for a new one. Not in anger, but only to safeguard the true. To safeguard it everywhere...I see him standing there over his plumb bob which never lies and never lies and the plumb bob is pointing motionless to the unimaginable center of the earth four thousand miles beneath his feet. Pointing to a blackness unknown and unknowable both in truth and in principle where God and matter are locked in a collaboration that is silent nowhere in the universe and it is this that guides him as he places one stone over two and two over one as did his fathers before him and his sons to follow and let the rain carve them if it can."[1]

Ben then talks about seeing samples of Papaw's work, some of it 80 years old, while driving in the region. "...in a thousand structures I've never seen a misplaced stone...The beauty of those structures would appear to be just a sort of a by-product, something fortuitous, but of course it is not. The aim of the mason was to make the wall stand up and that was his purpose in its entirety. The beauty of the stonework is simply a reflection of the purity of the mason's intention."[1]

Papaw and Ben feel a passionate responsibility to their profession and for its integrity. They believe what they do matters not only for the quality of the wall they build, which can be seen by all, but also for what cannot be seen, what almost no one will know or understand or value. They do things right out of respect for their profession, their craft and most of all, out of respect for themselves. The characters that disdain such values, Big Ben and Soldier, are chronically unhappy and unfulfilled and find it hard to love unconditionally. They make excuses for their unhappiness, their impatience and the short-cuts taken in their work and in their lives. For them, too, their jaded and cynical views of work are of one piece with their views of life.

The message is clear: Integrity in one's work and a passion for doing the right thing and doing things right are an inseparable part of what we love and value, of what brings happiness. Medicine is the same. Doing the work that we love is a privilege and a blessing; doing it with the same integrity and passion for truth as Papaw is the way we respect our patients, our profession, and ourselves.

25 June 2006

Reference
[1] McCarthy C: *The Stonemason: A Play in Five Acts.* New York, NY. Ecco, 1994

MEDICAL ETHICS AND VALUES

Client Billing and Self-Referral

IN THE 30 SEPTEMBER 2005 ISSUE of *The Wall Street Journal*, David Armstrong reported on "client billing" by physicians.[1] Client billing works like this: a dermatologist does a skin biopsy and sends the specimen to a pathology lab for analysis. The lab has previously struck a deal with the dermatologist to charge him $25 to examine a skin biopsy. The dermatologist then charges the insurance company or the patient $100 for the test.

So the client for the test, the dermatologist, has billed for a professional exam he did not perform. Keep in mind that he has already charged for seeing the patient and obtaining the biopsy and the pathology lab has already provided free mailing kits for the sample. So the dermatologist makes a $75 profit on each biopsy for doing no work. It is one of the many forms of fee-splitting, a practice that the American Medical Association condemns. Client billing is illegal when seeking reimbursement from Medicare. It is not allowed in some states and by some health insurers, like Blue Cross Blue Shield of Georgia. However, it is not illegal in most states when billing most insurers or when taking direct payment from the patient.

Where client billing is illegal, artificial structures have been set up to meet the letter of the law, while violating its intent. One such mechanism described by Armstrong is the "condo" lab within a building that houses condo labs for many practices. For example, the dermatologist mentioned above could buy or rent space in a building fitted for the purpose and buy the necessary equipment to outfit it (this building could be anywhere). The doctor then pays a management fee to a lab company that does the tests in his lab room and pays a pathologist per case for a professional diagnosis; the doctor then bills the payer. Since the doctor owns the facility, he believes he can legally bill Medicare for the services. (The inspector general of the Department of Health and Human Services believes, however, that this may violate anti-kickback laws.)

Just so dermatologists don't feel singled out, Armstrong reports similar deals by gastroenterologists who collect a large number of biopsies endoscopically; the same practice can be found among some urologists and gynecologists.

These practices disturb some physicians, including pathologists. I received a copy of a report to the College of American Pathologists by one of its members, pointing out his concern and that of many of his colleagues. These pathologists believe client billing to be unethical, wasteful, and medically dangerous. They say it is unethical because it is fee-splitting, which means being paid just for sending business to someone without having any professional input, and it means charging the payer a hidden fee, while the payer assumes that the charge is for the service provided.

They say it is wasteful because there is clear evidence that self-referral leads to over-utilization of these lab tests. There are reports of dermatologists who routinely remove 10 or 15 skin lesions from a patient, half of which are 2 mm or less in greatest dimension. These practitioners do five- to tenfold the number of biopsies of the average for dermatologists in the region. Although this is undoubtedly an extreme example, it underscores the temptation to do what is medically unnecessary to make a profit. Pathologists have told me of similar examples of the inflation of billing for biopsies by urologists.

And they also say client billing can be dangerous. Armstrong reports that one of the labs that offers such deals was banned from doing business in California because it operated "in a manner which poses a threat of injury to public health."[1] It seems that this lab was hiring pathologists and asking them to examine far more samples than was safe or reasonable by commonly accepted standards. Clearly, when charging $20 or $25 to analyze a biopsy, the lab must churn out results at a very high rate to make a profit with as few personnel as possible. Because of a lawsuit, it came to light that one pathologist in this banned company had quit after only 6 months because the workload was so great as to be unsafe and affected the quality patient care, and because the volume of work exhausted her. In a well-publicized case, deeply discounted pathology services for Pap smears led to the death of women several years ago due to poor quality.

Although client billing is spreading rapidly and federal authorities seem helpless to do anything about non-Medicare-Medicaid billing, a similar and, arguably, more serious and widespread problem is self-referral. A major example of this practice was reported in detail by Drs. David Levin and Vijay Rao in an article entitled, "Turf Wars in Radiology: The Over-Utilization of Imaging Resulting from Self-Referral."[2] Self-referral means referring patients to facilities or services in which the referring physician has equity or other financial interest. Here are quotes from the article that describe the issues.

"A recent report by the Medicare Payment Advisory Commission [MedPAC] to Congress indicated that the utilization of diagnostic imaging is growing more rapidly than that of any other type of physician service. This has engendered concern among those who pay for health care. In this article, the authors review the role of self-referral in driving up imaging utilization.

"A number of studies of the self-referral factor in imaging have been conducted over the past three decades. These have consistently shown that when non-radiologist physicians operate their own imaging equipment and have the opportunity to self-refer, their utilization is substantially higher than among other physicians who refer their patients to radiologists. It has also been shown that the vast bulk of the recent increases in imaging utilization are attributable to non-radiologists who self-refer. The authors estimate that the cost to the American health care system of unnecessary imaging resulting from self-referral by non-radiologists is $16 billion per year.

"In March 2003... a MedPAC report...reviewed growth in Medicare services between 1999 and 2002 in four broad categories: evaluation and management (E&M), procedures, tests, and imaging. Average annual growth during that period was 1.8% for E&M services, 4.1% for procedures, and 5.6% for tests, but it was 9,0% for imaging. Anecdotal evidence from the commercial health care insurance sector suggests recent rapid growth in the utilization of imaging there as well."[2]

The authors go on to describe comparative studies which showed that self-referral resulted in 1.7 to 7.7 times greater use of imaging studies for the same conditions compared to referral to other radiologists. This effect is not limited to diagnostic imaging. The General Accounting Office, an arm of Congress, analyzed millions of office visits in Florida and found that self-referring physicians used 1.95 and 5.13 times as many diagnostic tests as those who referred patients to radiologists.

Another study cited in the article looks at "Utilization trends for all Medicare non-invasive diagnostic imaging between 1993 and 1999 compared radiologists and non-radiologists. Among radiologists during that six-year interval, the procedure utilization rate per thousand Medicare beneficiaries dropped by 4%, whereas the relative value unit (RVU) rate per thousand increased by 7%. The RVU rate is a better measure of workload and the complexity of services. By comparison, among non-radiologists, the procedure utilization rate increased by 25%, and the RVU rate increased by 32%. In essence, this means that the vast bulk of the increases in imaging utilization rates, workload, and billings in recent years are attributable to non-radiologists."[2]

And finally, a study of "The test-ordering behavior of a group of 15 primary care physicians in a for-profit ambulatory care center in Boston before and after a financial incentive plan was introduced. Before the plan, the physicians were paid a straight salary; after the plan was instituted, they could earn bonuses based on revenues they generated for the center. The facility had on-site radiographic equipment, and referring patients to it was one way the physicians could generate more revenue. Their utilization of radiology was compared during a winter three-month period before the incentive plan was instituted and the same three-month period a year later, after it had gone into effect. During the latter period, 11 of the 15 physicians ordered more x-rays, and overall utilization by the entire group increased by 16%."

One might argue that pathologists and radiologists are angry that they are losing business or income from these financial practices, and that may be so. But the evidence suggests that the more important issues are ethics, waste, and danger. Both client billing and self-referral are devices that create financial incentives that: can lead to profiteering and increased utilization of tests; provide no demonstrable benefit for the patient; add substantially to the cost of health care; and decrease the efficiency and quality of care. Some steps have been taken to control or eliminate these practices, but the response from the professional societies has been more like a whisper than a roar. Burying proclamations in largely unread "ethical guidelines" does not suggest that these practices are a major concern, despite the fact that they fray the fabric of our profession.

As medical professionals we receive special trust and respect from society because of our training, expertise, and our commitment of personal responsibility for the good of our patients and for the public good. If we allow the basis of that trust to be eroded, our profession becomes a trade and our exceptional place in society will be unjustified; we then become just another commercial vendor out to make an extra buck.

25 November 2005

References

[1] Armstrong D: How some doctors turn a $79 profit from a $30 test. *The Wall Street Journal*, September 30, 2005

[2] Levin DC, Rao VM: Turf wars in radiology: The over-utilization of imaging resulting from self-referral. *J Am Coll Radiol* 1:169-172, 2004

MEDICAL ETHICS AND VALUES

Are We Single Agents, Double Agents, or Free Agents?

CONSIDER THE FOLLOWING QUOTE:
"Traditionally, physicians have acted as [single] agents advocating for the patients best interests, conforming to familiar professional ethics and societal expectations. With commercial managed care's growth and emphasis on cost control, health plans began imposing restrictions on physician's autonomy. Physicians often found themselves playing the role of "double agents," with potentially conflicting responsibilities to patients and insurers. Now in the post-managed care era, physicians have responded to mounting financial pressures with a range and intensity of activities that evoke images of "free agents" defending their own financial interests and challenge established professional norms."[1]

The quote is from a 2004 article, "Financial Pressures Spur Physician Entrepreneurism," by Pham, et al., in *Health Affairs*.[1] The article is one of a pair by the authors that is introduced by an editorial prologue, "Challenges for Physician Practice."[2]

The trends described in these articles will be familiar to oncologists, including: declining reimbursement for traditional physician services that is often not remedied by increasing volume; declining physician autonomy; the growth of physician investment in non-traditional income sources that provide more generous reimbursement; and the growth of single-specialty practices that have greater economic power.

The authors used cardiology and orthopedics surveys to illustrate these points. Physicians surveyed favored: increasing the volume of services over competing on efficiency or quality; increasing prices for services; and retreating from less lucrative services, e.g., declining to care for Medicaid or Medicare patients.

I would add a more worrisome trend – making major medical decisions that appear to be primarily for economic gain. An example of this slippery slope was reported on the front page of *The New York Times*.[3] It described increasingly heavy use of aggressive interventions such as coronary angioplasty and the insertion of stents for partially occluded vessels at a time when major studies show that heart attacks are not prevented by these procedures.

An interventional cardiologist from the University of Texas Southwestern in Dallas provides a quote from the trenches of daily practice. "If you're an invasive cardiologist and Joe Smith, the local internist, is sending you patients, and if you tell them that they don't need the procedure, pretty soon Joe Smith doesn't send patients anymore. Sometimes you can talk yourself into doing it even though in your heart of hearts you don't think its right." The same cardiologist explained the enthusiasm for the aggressive procedures thus: "I think it is ingrained in the American psyche that the worth of medical care is directly related to how aggressive it is. Americans want a full court press."[3] Although that public attitude is common in my experience as well, taking medical action on that basis blames the patient and dodges personal and professional responsibility. If there were no economic incentive to do the invasive procedure, what would the cardiologist recommend and actually carry out?

But what struck me most profoundly were two words in the article by Pham: "free agents."[1] Has it come to this? Are the authors and many finger-pointing payers right? Has the rationale for care by medical specialists, oncologists included, evolved from a philosophy of, "what is best for the patient comes first," to straddling the lines between the often contradictory needs and desires of patient and payer, professional ethics, and personal economics? And has the rationale finally now come to behaving primarily as animals in an economic jungle seriously concerned only with *numero uno*?

It is impossible to deny that there are physicians who behave as if the patient serves principally as a source of revenue, whose practices are focused inordinately on the business of medicine. They are the "free agents" described in Pham's article.[1] More specifically, one might call them "econo-docs," those who practice economics first and the "doc" part last.

These trends have more to do with oncology than we would hope. I will address the implications for oncology in my next essay.

25 April 2004

References

[1] Pham HH, Kevers KJ, May JH, et al: Financial pressures spur physician entrepreneurism. *Health Affairs* 23:70-80, 2004

[2] Prologue: Challenges for physician practice. *Health Affairs* 23:69, 2004

[3] Kolata G: New heart studies question the value of opening arteries. *The New York Times*, March 21, 2004

MEDICAL ETHICS AND VALUES

Econo-Docs in Oncology

I HAVE PREVIOUSLY CITED STUDIES (*see pp 163-164*) that described the evolution of medical specialists from acting as "single agents" (for the patient), to "double agents" (for patient and payer), and now to "free agents" (for themselves). I called the free agents "econo-docs," for whom economics comes first and the doc part last. And now I ask: Are we oncologists like the interventional cardiologists and orthopedists cited in the articles?[1-3]

It is impossible to deny that there are some of us in oncology who behave as if the patient serves principally as a source of revenue and whose practices are focused inordinately, and sometimes obscenely, on the business of medicine. I have spoken with numerous oncologists who can provide examples of (other) oncologists who fit the profile of the "econo-docs."

Econo-docs engage in behavior that is unprofessional at best and mired in unethical conflicts of interest at worst. A few examples of such behavior follow: prescribing chemotherapy that is futile ("churning"); prescribing expensive agents, like erythropoietin, without justification based on established guidelines; prescribing chemotherapy that the oncologist sells to the patient at an exorbitant markup; ordering outpatients to receive costly intravenous hydration that is not indicated; using software programs to choose among drugs not by relative efficacy and safety, but by highest profit margin; and preferentially referring patients to other specialty services in which they personally hold equity positions that are hidden from the patient and public, e.g., radiation oncology or diagnostic imaging facilities.

Other examples include responding to the pending decline in chemotherapy reimbursement by sending to their patients frightening letters that threaten the use of inferior or more toxic therapy, or indicating to their Medicare patients that they may no longer be cared for.[4,5] An informal survey of community medical oncology practices revealed that top incomes in a practice often exceed $1,000,000, particularly in large practices in smaller metropolitan areas.

To be sure, health maintenance organizations, Medicare, and medical insurance companies have created a perverse system of reimbursement The system values an appendectomy more than spending hours establishing and telling a cancer patient the diagnosis and prognosis, laying out the treatment options, talking to the family, and repeating information that the often stunned and distraught patient cannot remember from one visit to the next. The system has also rewarded oncologists far more handsomely for the purchase and resale of chemotherapy than for face-to-face care of the patient. Yes, the system's incentives are terribly warped. But with few exceptions, the outcry of the oncology community at the unjust reimbursement schedule came only after the lucrative chemotherapy business was threatened.

Should we respond that these econo-docs make up a minority of cancer care-givers and, therefore, should not concern us? Should we ignore them as minor aberrations that one is likely to find in any profession? Or tolerate them as overzealous business types who occasionally step over the line of ethical propriety? "Boys will be boys?" Well, let me test the reader's response with related questions.

Is the reader outraged at rapacious business leaders' theft of billions of dollars from ordinary people, while lying and cheating to hide their crimes? That chief executive officers/chairmen vote themselves almost unimaginably rich compensation packages as their companies consistently lose value? That cozy complicity in these shenanigans is practiced by certified public accountants? I am outraged and I hope the reader is. One might argue that these professionals committed more serious breaches than the econo-docs and that some were engaged in criminal activity.

But the concern here is not for legality, but the much higher standard of professional ethics. As professionals who are entrusted with the care of the sick and who take an oath of ethical behavior, we are held to much higher standards because we care for people at very vulnerable and often dangerous periods of their lives. The behavior of econo-docs has exposed major cracks in professional ethical norms that include actual or potential conflicts of interest.

Most of all, by taking advantage of vulnerable patients, econo-docs betray the public trust; that is what should concern us most of all.

It is true that there are some scoundrels in every profession. But the bigger worry is that our silent tolerance, and sometimes admiration, of the econo-docs' entrepreneurial activities may insidiously encourage some of the large majority to cross the line and engage in practices devised primarily for economic gain. The irony is that econo-docs most likely will find a way to prosper under the Medicare Modernization Act of 2003; it is the more non-entrepreneurial docs that are likely to suffer most and even be forced out of business.

While an ethical profession may be embarrassed by the transgressions of the few, the quiet acquiescence, approval, and participation of the many ordinary, basically decent docs eventually destroys its professional fabric.

Just because our patients like us and trust us does not necessarily mean we give high-quality care that is free of economic conflicts of interest. It is the professional responsibility of each of us and of our leaders to be vigilant and take steps to assure ourselves that both, in fact, are so.

10 May 2004

References

[1] Pham HH, Kevers KJ, May JH, et al: Financial pressures spur physician entrepreneurism. *Health Affairs* 23:70-80, 2004

[2] Prologue: Challenges for physician practice. *Health Affairs* 23:69, 2004

[3] Kolata G: New heart studies question the value of opening arteries. *The New York Times*, March 21, 2004

[4] Harris G: Among cancer doctors, a Medicare revolt: New payment system spurs talk of return to hospital care and old drugs. *The New York Times*, March 11, 2004

[5] Editorial: Cancer care tactics. *The New York Times*, March 22, 2004

MEDICAL ETHICS AND VALUES

The Role of a Professional Society in Medical Ethics – 1

I HAVE SERVED ON THE ETHICS COMMITTEE of the American Society of Clinical Oncology (ASCO) and spent a lot of time reading and trying to understand the ethical issues and what role ASCO might or should play.

My first Ethics Committee meeting was focused on oncologists' relationship with the pharmaceutical industry. As the chairman pointed out, that is the hot issue of the day. This is certainly a critically important issue because oncologists and the pharmaceutical industry need each other. The National Cancer Institute once was the major source of new anti-cancer agents, but that has not been true for 20 years or more, so we must depend on industry. The industry obviously needs us to test new agents and to prescribe them. So a productive, ethically sound relationship is in all of our interests.

In addition, I believe there are other important ethical issues facing oncologists, particularly in their relationships with patients, medical colleagues, and with payers, including governments. I will touch on only a few points for this essay and hope to cover others in the future.

Few people would condone actual conflicts of interest, such as prescribing a very expensive intravenous drug that brings lucrative reimbursement instead of a more effective and inexpensive oral drug. But what if the cheap drug is just equally effective and also is given parenterally? The only significant difference then is cost and reimbursement. Is that an actual or potential conflict of interest? If potential, how is one to avoid a decision biased only toward better reimbursement?

If an oncologist receives non-medical gifts from a pharmaceutical representative of small monetary value, is that any type of conflict of interest? If a patient were told, would the patient perceive a conflict of interest? And if there were evidence of that perceived conflict, should the physician refrain from accepting any gift, or meals, or donuts for journal club?

Some of these issues have been addressed in a pair of articles in the *New England Journal of Medicine*, which I strongly recommend.[1,2] David Blumenthal reviews the evidence showing that gifts do influence decisions in favor of the gift giver, even if unconsciously. Furthermore, neither the size of the gift nor whether it is of a medical nature seems to make a difference; the influence remains. Also, patients are far more likely to perceive a conflict of interest than the physician, regardless of the type or monetary value of the gift. In fact, those who receive the most gifts are least likely to believe there may be a conflict of interest.[1]

In the second article, by David Studdert and colleagues, the title says it all, "Financial Conflicts of Interest in Physicians' Relationships with the Pharmaceutical Industry—Self Regulation in the Shadow of Federal Prosecution."[2] In short, steps are being taken by industry and the medical profession to address conflicts of interest, but only after government legislation put the heat on them with the threat of even more government intervention. The authors observe that compared to 4 years ago, the current amount of regulatory, self-regulatory and prosecutorial activity is remarkably high. They believe government will continue to press on this issue because of the evidence that even small gratuities influence physician behavior and because the cost of drugs to Medicare has gone through the roof; thus, this effort has a cost-cutting as well as an ethical rationale.

The authors quote critics who are skeptical that guidelines produced by the American Medical Association or other professional organizations can be effective, partly because surveys show that most physicians believe it is okay to accept free drug samples, gifts, and other gratuities of modest value (dollar limit not specified), and partly because there is no detection or enforcement mechanism.

Now back to my main issue: What can ASCO do to promote the ethical behavior of oncologists and what should the Ethics Committee try to get ASCO to do? I shall describe a few possibilities and some obstacles to effective action.

First, as a professional association, ASCO can provide guidance for the highest ethical behavior in three ways: by its own example, by offering guidelines and by education. However, since a majority of ASCO'S revenue for providing services to its members and for fellowships to investigators comes from the pharmaceutical industry, it is not in a strong position to provide credible guidance on avoiding conflicts of interest with industry. ASCO has developed extensive guidelines for avoiding conflicts of interest for its officers and for commercial exhibitors at its meetings, but I know of no data on their effectiveness. ASCO could make its use of pharmaceutical company monies more transparent to the rank and file and to the public, perhaps providing an annual, detailed accounting in the *Journal of Clinical Oncology*.

I don't know if these or other measures would be sufficient to provide ASCO the moral authority necessary to play a meaningful role in addressing conflicts of interest but, in my view, it would be important to make the attempt.

Second, ASCO can provide ethical guidance for the physician-patient relationship with special emphasis on areas prominent in oncology. For example, when is it appropriate to give second- or third- or fourth-line therapy that is of no known value for controlling the patient's cancer? Never? When the patient or family wants to "try anything?" Only in a clinical trial? Are fee-splitting and self-referral (e.g., to a facility or service in which the physician has a financial interest unknown to the patient) ever acceptable? I am unaware that ASCO has a position on issues such as these.

Third, ASCO can provide the oncologist with tools to blunt the unfortunate effects of the multi-billion dollar marketing blitz by the industry. For example, how should one deal with patients who bring false hopes or request inappropriate therapy after seeing on television direct-to-patient advertising for prescription drugs. This would be an example of pointing the finger at ourselves, of taking responsibility.

My point, and strongly held belief, is that even if ASCO and its members were to have no actual conflicts of interest, it is best for both to recognize and avoid potential and perceived conflicts, as well. This is one way to earn and deserve patients' trust, the bedrock of the physician-patient relationship.

It would be naïve to believe that any of these suggestions, as well as other, perhaps better approaches, would lead to the elimination of conflicts of interest. We are, after all, human beings controlled by human nature. But it is the duty of a professional medical society to espouse and promulgate ideals of professional behavior. Perfection is not a reasonable goal, but education and improvement are.

25 November 2004

References
[1] Blumenthal D: Doctors and drug companies. *N Engl J Med* 351:1885-1890, 2004
[2] Studdert DM, Mello MM, Brennan TA: Financial conflicts of interest in physicians' relationships with the pharmaceutical industry–self-regulation in the shadow of federal prosecution. *N Engl J Med* 351:1891-1900, 2004

The Role of a Professional Society in Medical Ethics – 2

IN A PREVIOUS ESSAY (see pp 168-170), I indicated that I have served on the American Society of Clinical Oncology (ASCO) Ethics Committee. I asked the readers to comment on any problems, positions or actions that the committee or ASCO should address. I received a number of responses by e-mail and had oral conversations with others. The responses were varied and thoughtful. I will group them under several headings, though some of the responses overlap the categories.

A Lack of Transparency
This was a recurring theme in most of the responses, which included a variety of examples that illustrate the concerns:

The academic physician pushes a particular regimen in a protocol while serving on the speakers' bureau of the pharmaceutical company (or receiving consulting fees) that has a financial stake in the outcome. Do the patients know that he/she has a financial relationship with the company? The academic oncologist receives research grants from industry for doing studies of its drugs or equipment. Does the patient know of this payment? The community oncologist has an ownership interest in a PET scanner to which he/she refers patients. Does the patient know this? Do the patients know that as a group, physicians with ownership in such facilities are more likely to order the test? One reader was concerned that chairs of ASCO committees that make practice recommendations might be paid speakers of a company. Does the ASCO leadership know and condone this and, if so, is this indicated in any written deliberations of the committee?

Pushing Regimens with No Significant Clinical Advantage
Some responders believe academic "thought leaders" recommend new (and more expensive) regimens that offer little or no practical advantage; they attribute this to incentives such as academic advancement, research grants, and speaker or consulting fees. Examples were offered such as "dose dense" regimens that require growth factors costing an additional $5,000 a month or more. "Not surprisingly," one responder wrote, "many of the

authors' smiling faces are on the numerous throwaway 'journalets' that I get, unsolicited...there is a huge perception of 50-something academic oncologists' 'cashing in' on honoraria with these trials. ASCO is still dominated by full-time academic oncologists, and each year more of them are on this gravy train."

Another respondent was concerned at the potential conflict of interest in phase 1 studies. "Are the patients clearly aware of the small benefits or are they simply told that 'there is no guarantee that you will receive any benefit from this drug?' When you think about it: if that [patient] enrolls, the person least likely to benefit is the patient and he/she endures all the toxicity (the institution, the physician, society, and the drug company all benefit)."

And another described a concern closer to home: "Your patient is diagnosed with metastatic ovarian cancer. Standard therapy would be taxol and carboplatin every 3 weeks. You and your staff are very familiar with the toxicity and efficacy of this regimen. You notice a new regimen of weekly taxol and carboplatin in a phase II study. Efficacy seems reasonable, and there might be some quality of life advantages. At your last practice meeting your fellow physicians note that with questionable reimbursement for the coming years, you need to maximize chemotherapy and nursing utilization to support all of the unpaid things we do like research and social and dietary help. You think: how can it hurt to give her weekly therapy? We get paid more so we can continue to be a good cancer center, the regimen will likely work reasonably well. Should the patient be aware of this thought process?"

Futile Chemotherapy and Poor End-of-Life Care
This is best described by one of the respondents who speaks for several other responders. "In the community I see major problems with end-of-life care of patients with cancer, willful blindness to the obvious failure of curative interventions to make a meaningful difference. [I see a] failure of advanced care planning, truth telling, and goal-setting, all of which have ethical content. In my former academic role I observed that phase I trials were presented dishonestly and proffered in lieu of appropriate end-of-life care (in order to avoid "difficult" conversations). As a result a lot of dying patients are getting futile care in the ICU at the point of death. Institutional review boards (IRBs) are great for looking at the scientific content of protocols but should be conjoined with an autonomous ethics IRB to assure dispassionate ethical review of clinical trials (matching risks and benefits)."

The Role of ASCO
Some respondents wondered how ASCO would fare in an independent analysis of its professional ethics, of its actual or apparent conflicts of interest. They believed ASCO should get its own house in order before telling others how to behave. One responder

recommended that the ASCO Ethics Committee have an independent ethicist(s) and/or independent community representatives as members; persons with no relationship to ASCO, its members or its benefactors. This responder apparently believes someone from a patient advocacy group is part of the establishment because of financial support from or social integration in the oncology establishment and would not qualify.

Another suggestion is that the *Journal of Clinical Oncology* should encourage and publish more papers on professional ethics that deal with specific oncology issues. Finally, one responder thought it was unethical for ASCO to put so little effort into public health oncology: he pointed out that reducing smoking has had far more benefit than many Gleevecs might and hepatitis vaccine has been a far more powerful tool for dealing with liver cancer than all the surgery and chemotherapy.

My conclusions from this exercise are that, in general, oncologists are well aware of some potential and actual ethical violations and professional conflicts of interest. Most see the problem in others and everyone I talked to was ready to offer an opinion or an example of unethical behavior by someone else, though it might be someone in their own practice group. So I believe that this is somewhat like the proverbial turd in the punchbowl–everyone sees it there, but nobody at the party wants to do something about it.

Respondents believe that ASCO has an important role to play in professional ethics. I agree and I have outlined several possible ways of fulfilling this responsibility in the last essay on the topic (*see pp 168-170*).

25 February 2005

MEDICAL ETHICS AND VALUES

Oncology Professional Meetings: Too Big? Too Commercial?

THE ANNUAL MEETINGS of the American Society of Clinical Oncology (ASCO) have huge successes by many measures. However, some attendees grouse about the meeting being too large and unwieldy or too commercial with its huge exhibit area and pervasive presence of industry. We shall address each of these questions after looking at some facts. These issues apply to other oncology professional meetings such as the annual meetings of the American Association of Cancer Research (AACR) and the American Society of Hematology (ASH) (and many other medical meetings).

Attendance by decade since ASCO's first meeting has been: 50 in 1964; 1,200 in 1974; 5,085 in 1984; 10,500 in 1994; 28,000 in 2004; and 32,000 in 2007. The largest 2-year increase was from 19,700 in 1999 to 26,500 in 2001. ASCO began managing its own annual meeting in 1998. The 28,000 attendees in 2004 included 21,000 professionals and 5,000 exhibitors, 49% domestic attendees and 51% internationals representing 104 countries. ASCO members made up 32% (8,960) and non-members 68% of attendees. Of the 21,614 ASCO members, 41.5% attended. One can safely assume that the same percentages apply to subsequent meetings. Nearly 3,000 abstracts are presented orally or by poster and scientific sessions are approaching 100 with at least twice as many educational sessions.

Too Big?

As a member of ASCO for 35 years, I find the meeting more difficult to negotiate due to the longer distances and overwhelmingly large program. I know many fewer attendees than I did; I may see few if any familiar faces during a stroll through the crowded corridors. In the old days, most members were American academics; they are now a minority. Also, I could easily attend virtually any session or get to single talks at several simultaneous sessions, flitting from one to another. Today it is very hard to change venues to catch a single presentation elsewhere due to the distances.

But I ask myself how much of this change is bad for our patients and attendees? Despite my curmudgeonly grumbles now and then, I think the growth has been inevitable and fortunate because oncology itself has grown in size, complexity and diversity at least as rapidly as ASCO. Oncology in Europe and parts of Asia and Latin America has grown robustly and the presence of those investigators, practitioners and trainees at the meeting enriches the meeting's ambience and furthers its mission to advance clinical oncology. The annual meeting provides a key, handy venue for unofficial side meetings because attendance is so high.

So I conclude that the size can be a mechanical handicap but, all in all, the growth in the program, attendance, and diversity has been a positive trend.

Furthermore, ASCO now offers smaller meetings around the country throughout the year that focus on a single cancer or issue. Such smaller, focused meetings organized by the AACR have been very popular and financially successful for many years. With an attendance of 100-300, the meetings encourage more interaction of attendees, many of whom have specific research or clinical interests in the narrower topic. Regional meetings, such as the "Best of ASCO" follow-ups, some under the auspices of state or regional ASCO affiliates, bring presentations closer to home. These smaller meetings often draw those who do not attend the annual meeting. Over the years, I have often found smaller workshop-style meetings more useful scientifically.

Too Commercial?
Some former presidents of ASCO and others have openly expressed concern that the annual meeting has become too commercial. They point to the "mind-blowing" commercial exhibits sponsored by pharmaceutical companies, some of which cost millions of dollars to stage, as an "obscene sales pitch" that demeans the meeting. Pharmaceutical companies also fund large, and some say extravagant, social events.

The critics also say that the substantial revenue that ASCO receives for leasing space to exhibitors is a bargain with the devil. They believe the revenue is seductive and becomes difficult to give up once staffing and programs become dependent on it, and that it risks allowing revenue to drive the growth of programs and staff rather than the reverse. Pharmaceutical companies also fund the travel to the annual meeting of a large proportion of international attendees. In fact, the annual meeting can now be held only in a few cities partly because of the hotel space now required, but also because there are few venues that have sufficient commercial exhibit space to meet the demand. Finally, the critics point to the fact that over 80% all ASCO's revenues comes from firms that sell cancer products.

In response, ASCO is working hard to reduce its reliance on such revenues, in particular by forming The ASCO Foundation, a separate non-profit organization charged with raising revenue for ASCO's educational and research programs. The hope is that non-profit philanthropic organizations might be more approachable by The Foundation. (Full disclosure–I have been a member of the Foundation's Board of Directors.) Of course, the membership must also support The Foundation if it is to succeed; philanthropies often ask how much the membership contributes to gauge its commitment to the mission.

ASCO also points out that it has put in place a stringent conflict of interest policy to reduce the likelihood of undue influence of commercial interests on the program and conduct of the annual meeting. Pharmaceutical companies provide unrestricted funds for fellowships and grants that are given by ASCO through a peer review process; this is viewed as an especially important use of such funds by ASCO leaders.

So is the meeting too commercial? Many people I talk to are either indifferent or say that commercial ties are inevitable in today's environment. Others, many with levels of integrity, experience and wisdom that demand respect, say it is an insidious, serious and growing problem. They believe that the mere fact that so much of ASCO's overall revenue (and travel funds for many oncologists, especially internationals) comes from pharmaceutical companies gives, at the very least, the appearance of a conflict of interest and that the elaborate exhibits serve no useful purpose other than to sell products and create a circus-like atmosphere at the meeting.

In my own case, I have gone back and forth on industry largesse in my career, mainly over small potatoes. I gladly accepted free baby formula and antibiotic samples for my kids when I was a house officer with a serious cash-flow problem. I have objected to drug company representatives buying coffee and donuts for tumor boards; I prevailed once and was voted down once. Some of the exhibits at the annual meeting are grotesque imitations of Las Vegas, but I do take an occasional cappuccino there. On a larger scale and qualitatively different from rentals of exhibit space, for 18 years I was an associate editor of the *Journal of Clinical Oncology* (JCO), which cannot be published without revenues from ads placed by pharmaceutical companies; I never felt any influence on my decisions from industry.

In fact, the ASCO annual meeting (and the JCO) as constituted today cannot be supported by membership dues and registration fees alone. To offer the services ASCO now provides with dues and fees alone would either be impossible or place an unacceptable burden on members and attendees.

My position on this matter is a tad idealistic with a large dose of pragmatism. I am uneasy, though not opposed, to ASCO's accepting money from industry for worthwhile programs–such a relationship can be mutually beneficial without the loss of integrity by either party. I think virtually all attendees understand that the exhibits and sponsored fellowships are not an endorsement of any product by ASCO.

However, I have a number of concerns. The first is for the very large absolute amount of industry support because it makes the stakes of the relationship so high. The second concern is that commercial funds make up such a large proportion of ASCO revenues that it gives the appearance of an improper or, at least, an unseemly relationship. Finally, dependence on the above may inevitably lead to a compelling need for ASCO to sustain and grow that level of support; like any addiction, will it someday be "at any cost?"

I see no short-term solution. So I offer a famous admonition to ASCO in this situation, "Eternal vigilance is the price of liberty." ASCO must be firm and very conservative in protecting the independence, scientific integrity, and propriety of the meeting. A formal assessment of the exhibits and of the annual financial transactions with industry by an independent group (non-ASCO members and non-physicians) would be prudent and helpful; sunshine can be an excellent antiseptic.

Expansion of the exhibit space for the sake of increasing revenue would be a dangerous step on a slippery slope. Programs, fellowships and grants should be evaluated as to their effectiveness, value, and appropriateness to ASCO's specific role; because not everything we do turns out well or remains effective and efficient, pruning should be formal and regular. As with cancer therapy, more is not necessarily better. Generating new programs and initiatives is easy; achieving and sustaining the highest quality is not.

The utter dependence of the annual meeting and other programs on pharmaceutical funds for their very existence is a foolish bet. A formal plan should be established to sustain the organization should a sudden reduction of such revenue reach 25%, 50% or more. The survival of ASCO without pharmaceutical revenues would be very difficult today; should ASCO bet that the money will always be there?

It is too soon to know whether The ASCO Foundation can raise enough revenue to forego a substantial portion of revenue from commercial sources; one worries that even if it does, those new revenues may simply add to rather than replace some portion of commercial revenues, leaving the proportion the same.

ASCO is healthy and productive. The JCO is doing extremely well both in its influence and finances, and the website and patient information services are of high quality. The meteoric growth of programs and staff has created a rich and powerful organization. But amid all the congratulatory back-slapping, ASCO should be careful not to lose its soul.

25 July 2004

MEDICAL ETHICS AND VALUES

Uncertainty and Ethics in Clinical Trials – 1

AN ARTICLE IN THE *BRITISH MEDICAL JOURNAL*[1] posed the following thesis: A randomized clinical trial (RCT) assumes that the outcome is not known or knowable with currently available knowledge (the "uncertainty principle"). If the outcome were known in advance, the trial would be unscientific and unethical. Therefore, to satisfy the uncertainty principle, in any large group of RCTs, the chance of demonstrating a better outcome for the control group or for the experimental group should be equal.

The authors tested this principle in a review of the RCTs of the Children's Oncology Group completed between 1955 and 1997. The meta-analysis included 126 trials and 36,567 patients. They found that the odds ratio for overall survival with experimental treatments was 0.96 (99% confidence interval of 0.89-1.03), meaning that the new treatments, on average, were as likely to be inferior as were the standard or control treatments. They also found that the result was not affected by publication bias, methodological quality, treatment type, disease, or comparator.

In an earlier study of adult oncology patients,[2] 93 randomized trials completed between 1981 and 1995 by two United States cooperative groups were similarly examined. They found that three studies favored the standard treatment, 70 favored neither, and 30 favored the experimental treatment. The average effect size was 1.20 (1.2 to 1 experimental over the standard treatment) with the 95% confidence range being 1.13-1.28.

The authors conclude that there was "a measurable average improvement in disease control associated with assignment to the experimental rather than the standard arm. However, the heterogeneity of outcomes and the small magnitude of advantage suggest that, as a group, these trials satisfy the uncertainty principle." Also, there was no apparent publication bias, i.e., non-publication of trials with negative results.[2]

A third study looked at similar parameters for trials sponsored by pharmaceutical companies.[3] The report, which was not limited to cancer studies, included 30 industry-sponsored trials and found that those trials were more likely to have outcomes favoring the industry sponsor's product than studies with other sponsors such as the National

Institutes of Health. The odds ratio was 4.05 (4.05 positive result in industry-sponsored to 1.0 in other sponsored trials) with a 95% confidence interval of 2.98-5.51. The authors conclude that, "Systematic bias favors products which are made by the company funding the research." The bibliography of the paper lists other studies that drew the same conclusion.

So we see a gradation of results that test the uncertainty principle. There clearly was no bias in the pediatric studies. Some bias was detected in the adult oncology studies, though not statistically significant enough to violate the uncertainty principle. And clear-cut bias was seen in the industry-sponsored trials.

There are a variety of explanations for these findings. One would expect large and very expensive RCTs sponsored by industry to be carefully chosen with "best bet" products. In other words, the dogs may have been screened out in phase 1 and phase 2 trials. Few novel front-line agents have been tested in pediatric RCTs in the past 30 years because pediatric oncology is not a lucrative business for the pharmaceutical industry. Consequently, most pediatric RCTs have tested variations of regimens using the same agents in both arms of a study in which the differences are likely to be small and there is no inherent pressure to favor one regimen over another. The result in non-industry trials for adult oncology patients is a bit in between; the small, but measurable bias may be due to the admixture of some hot new agents. Enthusiasm runs high in such instances since for adult oncology, new agents with substantial effectiveness were rare in the time periods under study.

There are less neutral explanations. It has been shown that industry trials are much less likely to be published, especially those with negative results. So there may be a publication bias that reduced the number of negative trials. It is also possible that biased studies have used inappropriate or inadequate controls. Another possibility explaining the bias is that the positive result, while statistically significant due to a very large study population, may be clinically unimportant. Approval of a new agent by the Food and Drug Administration is the pot of gold for the industry, so a good strategy would be to invest in a very large trial that requires a smaller difference in outcome from controls to achieve statistical significance.

These observations affirm the fact that industry-sponsored trials are far more likely to favor their products, and that the bias may be intentional or not, nefarious or not. But that begs the question of who should bear responsibility for the integrity of the trials. As a mentor once told me, you don't condemn lions for killing and eating zebras; that's what lions do for a living. Likewise, it is foolish to blame only industry for a bias toward their products; that's what businesses do for a living. Although I do not exonerate industry—many of their current practices are marginally or even frankly unethical, in my view.

But the focus should not be on industry, but on us, the oncologists who order the therapy and conduct the trials. Unlike the lions and the medical products industry, our training, professional culture, societal standing, and sentiments are all geared to helping and representing the interests of the patient. In that capacity, we are duty-bound to do our very best to avoid bias, particularly bias that results in personal financial gain, in assessing and prescribing diagnostics and treatments. So in the end, it is we who must be the guardians of that trust given to us by society in general and our patients in particular.

In my next essay, I will expand on this theme and discuss recent reports calling for more stringent rules for eliminating conflicts of interest.

10 March 2006

References

[1] Kumar A, Soares H, Wells B, et al: Are experimental treatments for cancer in children superior to established treatments? Observational study of randomised controlled trials by the Children's Oncology Group. *BMJ* 331:1295, 2005

[2] Joffe S, Harrington DP, George SL, et al: Satisfaction of the uncertainty principle in cancer clinical trials: Retrospective cohort analysis. *BMJ* 328:1463, 2004

[3] Lexchin J, Bero LA, Djulbegovic B, et al: Pharmaceutical industry support and research outcome and quality: Systematic review. *BMJ* 326:1167-1170, 2003

MEDICAL ETHICS AND VALUES

Uncertainty and Ethics in Clinical Trials – 2

IN MY PREVIOUS ESSAY (*see pp 178-180*), I discussed the potential for conflicts of interest in clinical trials. Using the uncertainty principle as the bedrock of randomized clinical trials, studies of large numbers of trials demonstrated no apparent bias in pediatric oncology trials since survival on average was just as likely to improve on the control therapy as on the experimental. There was some relatively insignificant bias in adult clinical trials run by cooperative groups, but significant bias in industry sponsored trials that favored the sponsors' product.

In light of the above, we examine recent reports that call for more stringent rules for eliminating conflicts of interest in academic medical centers. In a report by Brennan et al,[1] the authors state that current conflict of interest policies of government, industry, and physician groups are inadequate. They describe social science studies of gift giving and receiving that indicate that even trivial gifts have a measurable psychological effect on the recipient that inclines him/her positively toward the product or manufacturer.

They propose much more stringent regulations for academic medical centers that include banning all gifts of any dollar amount to physicians, banning pharmaceutical samples given directly to physicians, and refusing support from manufacturers, directly or indirectly, for continuing medical education programs or physician travel to meetings.

A second paper from Yale University describes the university's guidelines for interactions between clinical faculty and the pharmaceutical industry.[2] These new guidelines ban faculty from receiving any form of gift, meal, or free drug samples (for personal use) from industry. The guidelines increase disclosure and transparency and create "arms-length" structures for any relationships with the pharmaceutical industry, including industry-sponsored fellowships, educational activities at Yale, industry-sponsored symposia, and other activities. These guidelines were developed in consultation with representatives of the pharmaceutical industry.

These articles agree that academic medical centers should provide leadership and example in avoiding conflicts of interest and they agree that current guidelines are inadequate. But in both articles there is only passing mention of conflicts of interest in industry-sponsored research and clinical trials. This passing mention is notable because of the extensive and financially substantial relationships between academic investigators, both physicians and basic scientists, and the biotechnology and pharmaceutical industries.

The article by Brennan et al says it is okay to "accept grants for general support of research (no specific deliverable products) from pharmaceutical and device companies, provided the grants are not designated for use by specific individuals."[1] And they believe academic medical centers should post on their public access websites all consulting agreements and unconditional grants with industry. The Yale article simply requires disclosure to the department chair all financial interests with industry.[2]

It may be true that getting a pad of paper or a pen bearing a drug company logo may influence a physician's prescribing action; I don't know if that specific circumstance has been tested. Even if some influence has been shown, its magnitude is likely to be very small compared to the sea of other influences. But it is striking to me that the much more serious matter of influencing the outcome of clinical trials was not addressed in the same depth as pens and pads. The potential negative impact of a biased trial, whether conscious or not, is orders of magnitude greater and far more lasting.

I am not opposed to more stringent conflict of interest rules, especially when larger sums of money are involved, such as in lavish dinners, payment for serving on speakers' bureaus, or payment of travel to an industry-sponsored meeting. (If the pens and pads disappeared tomorrow from exhibits, most of us wouldn't notice.) But the ethical principles applied should include reasonableness and proportionality, meaning that the degree of stringency should be proportional to the risk and degree of harm caused by the violation.

I would put a 25-cent pen at one end of the gravitas scale and clinical trial bias at the other end. One runs the risk of burning too much fuel on minor issues leaving little for conflicts of interest with the potential for major violations of scientific ethical norms.

25 March 2006

References

[1] Brennan TA, Rothman DJ, Blank L, et al: Health industry practices that create conflicts of interest. JAMA 295:429-433, 2006

[2] Coleman DL, Kazdin AE, Miller LE, et al: Guidelines for Interactions between Clinical Faculty and the Pharmaceutical Industry: One Medical School's Approach. Acad Med 81:154-160, 2006

Chapter 6

LEADERSHIP IN MEDICINE

I have had a number of leadership positions with responsibility for medical staff and medical institutions. In the course of my career I became interested in what experts, and my own experience, have said about strong and effective leaders. These findings, of course, do not apply solely to medicine but also to most human endeavors.

What Makes a Great Leader?

SINCE CHANGES IN LEADERSHIP ARE UNDERWAY at the Food and Drug Administration (FDA) and the National Cancer Institute (NCI), two organizations that have a profound impact on oncology, this is an opportune time to ask what makes a good leader of these organizations and, better yet, what makes a great leader.

Leadership matters; it matters a lot. This is so whether the organization is a business, a practice, a hospital, an academic institution, or a government agency. Books on business success, including leadership, seem to be everywhere. Typical is the book by Jack Welch, the former chief executive office of General Electric, which became a best-seller.[1] Whereas books on leadership of non-profit organizations, particularly those in health sciences and health care, are almost non-existent, leadership qualities are shared in both venues. So let's review what some gurus of management have had to say on the subject.

One of my favorite sources of business management wisdom is Peter Drucker. This legendary sage understood and clearly described the features of running successful businesses. He is famous for believing that integrity and high ethical standards were central to good business practice because it was the right thing to do, but also because it was good for the long-term health of an organization. Here is an excerpt from his work.

"What would I look for in picking a leader of an institution? First, I would look at what the candidates have done, what their strengths are—you can only perform with strength—and what have they done with it? Second, I would look at the institution and ask: 'What is the one immediate key challenge?' I would try to match the strength with the needs. Then I would look for integrity. A leader sets an example, especially a strong leader."[2]

Drucker then quotes a famous and successful business leader whom he asked what he looked for in a leader. And the man responded, "I always ask myself, would I want one of my sons to work under that person? If [the leader] is successful…would I want my son to look like that?" Drucker then concludes, "This, I think, is the ultimate question."

He continues, "In human affairs, the distance between the leaders and the average is a constant. If leadership performance is high, the average will go up." And finally, "Effective leaders delegate, but they do not delegate the one thing that will set the standard. They do it."

This last principle was also held by another well known management expert, W. Edwards Deming, who is best known for being the American consultant who helped revitalized Japanese industry after the war. "It is the responsibility of management to discover the barriers that prevent workers from taking pride in what they do. Rather than helping workers do their job correctly, most supervisors don't know the work they supervise. They have never done the job."[3] Deming goes on to say that such supervisors often use numbers or quotas as the only basis for judgment, without understanding the nature of the work.

The greatest leader in American history was, in my view, Abraham Lincoln. This view was cemented by a recent book that focused on his leadership and political skills and, of course, on aspects of his personal character that shaped the former.[4] Lincoln's integrity, vision, and bedrock principles were combined with uncommon political skills acquired in his Illinois years, and with a keen sense of public opinion. These enabled him to navigate skillfully the most difficult and treacherous times of our country. He devoured information from all sources and sent aides into the field to obtain first-hand information which helped him make astute strategic decisions. He was an uncommon leader who engaged some political enemies in his administration because he believed they were the best people for the jobs.

In my experience, it has been clear that the ill effects of poor leadership, at any level from chief executive officer to department head to housekeeping, insidiously permeate an entire institution. This invariably leads to inefficiency at best, and at worst leads to falling dominoes of lost opportunity or catastrophe. Leadership matters even though its effectiveness may not be apparent in the short term. In fact, it is often most effective when its workings and angst are not apparent to most of the people most of the time.

What makes great leaders is not a secret. They not only have grace under pressure, which means both courage and character, they remain focused on the important aspects of an issue in the midst of chaos. Great leaders repeatedly articulate a consistent, simple public vision by example, conviction, and actions. If the troops don't know what is expected of them, what direction is set or what the leader values most, that is the leader's fault.

However, this vision must be backed by public acts, not just words. There are many opportunities to demonstrate one's vision, both subtle and overt. Whom the leader hires, fires, and promotes sends the most effective signal, but smaller acts can indirectly express his or her values. Great leaders take satisfaction in the success of team members and try to hire people who are better than they are.

I end with two qualities that help distinguish a great leader from a good leader, especially in the not-for-profit world. First, though he or she remains confident in final decisions, has humility in sufficient measure to mitigate arrogance, and promotes active listening to those holding other views. Second, he knows that at some time he will be asked to compromise basic principles. If personal values cannot be sustained, the great leader is prepared to lose favor, be fired, or quit over a key principle. If the position or stature or pay means so much that the leader will not put his job on the line for a core value, he is no longer free and has taken a step onto a slippery slope. Great leaders have the mindset upon taking a position of holding core values and principles dear, no matter what the cost.

25 April 2006

References

[1] Welch J with Byrne JA: *Jack: Straight from the gut*. New York, NY. Warner Books, 2001

[2] Drucker P: *The Essential Drucker: The Best of Sixty Years of Peter Drucker's Essential Writings on Management*. New York, NY. Harper Collins, 2001

[3] Walton M: *The Deming Management Method*. New York, NY. Putnum Publishing Group, 1986

[4] Carwardine R: Lincoln: *A Life of Purpose and Power*. New York, NY. Knopf, 2006

LEADERSHIP IN MEDICINE

Leadership of the Food and Drug Administration

IN MY LAST ESSAY (*see pp 184-186*), I used the changes in leadership underway at the Food and Drug Administration (FDA) and the National Cancer Institute (NCI) as an occasion for describing the characteristics of great leaders. I pointed out that there are personal and professional qualities that distinguish poor, good, and great leaders.

Here is a recap from that column on choosing effective leaders:
1. Has the candidate been an effective leader at another institution? Will he leave his current institution substantially better off than when he arrived?
2. Has he articulated a clear vision and rallied the troops behind him? Was this vision backed by public acts, not just words?
3. Has he hired strong, accomplished lieutenants and replaced the weak or incompetent?
4. Do his strengths meet the one immediate key challenge of his new institution?
5. Has he set an example by his integrity and humility?
6. Would I want my son or daughter to work for the candidate and be mentored by him?
7. Would he sacrifice his job for a core principle or is he welded to the party line?

Here I will deal with the FDA. Dr. Andrew von Eschenbach has been nominated by President Bush to head the FDA; at this writing, von Eschenbach has stepped down as director of the NCI to assume his new role. He heads the FDA in an interim capacity until his confirmation by the Senate. Dr. von Eschenbach has a public record from which cancer researchers may judge his effectiveness as director of the NCI; that may suggest how well he will be a good fit for the FDA position. The following comments were gleaned from conversations with about 75 cancer research leaders. The researchers all spoke to me with the understanding that they would not be identified. I have framed their comments as if in response to the seven questions above.
1. Effective leader of NCI? Did he leave the NCI better off than when he arrived? Opinions varied, but most believe he lost credibility with his pledge to "eliminate death and suffering from cancer by 2015," which was characterized as "magical think-

ing" since he never articulated specific short and long-term plans to achieve that goal.

Did he leave the NCI better off? The responses were nearly unanimous that he left the NCI worse off than when he arrived. The following is a characteristic comment. "He knew from the day he arrived that NCI was headed for a serious budget crunch, a situation he inherited. But he had four years to deal with it and failed to blunt the progressive constriction in funding of investigator-initiated grants. Instead of planning for the belt-tightening, money was spent on large, costly new programs at the expense of research project grants." Many, including three Nobel laureates who spoke at the recent American Association for Cancer Research meeting, said that a sustained pay line at current levels for research project grants will be catastrophic for the future of cancer research, with many young investigators—the seed corn of cancer research—leaving the field of creative discovery research.

2. Articulated clear vision? Rallied the troops? The 2015 vision was articulated repeatedly, but nobody believed it, so the troops—cancer scientists—did not follow because they could not understand how this would be accomplished. In public statements, Drs. Harold Varmus and Paul Nurse, both Nobel laureates and leaders of prestigious cancer research institutions, and others called the goal unreasonable.

3. Hired (or retained) strong lieutenants? Many believe that the departure of Drs. Barbara Rimer and Robert Wittes was a major loss from which the NCI still has not recovered. Some comments reflect the preponderance of opinion: "[Dr. Anna] Barker and [Dr. Mark] Clanton are not in the same league as Barbara and Bob when it comes to cancer research."

4. Strengths meet the needs of FDA? Many responded in the negative, while others said there were far more qualified people for the job, with more experience in drug development research. Many believe maintaining the scientific integrity and professionalism of the drug review process is the most important need. The general belief is that the Bush administration's priority was to prevent approval of the Plan B drug (the "morning after" pill to avert a pregnancy) and that was a major force in their selection of von Eschenbach.

5. Was he an example of integrity and humility? This response was also mixed. Some believe that, whatever his shortcomings, he did what he believed was right and stuck to it. Others questioned two of his activities, first reported in *The Cancer Letter*. First, serving as a board member of C-Change (formerly the National Dialogue on Cancer) along with leaders of the pharmaceutical industry was thought to create the appearance or potential of a conflict of interest. Also his appearance and voiced support at

political events for a Florida legislator, U.S. Representative E. Clay Shaw, running for re-election raised concerns. Some commented that the 2015 promise showed a lack of humility, an essential quality for leaders of organizations to gain and sustain excellence (see the best seller, "Good to Great" by Jim Collins[1]).

6. Would you want your son or daughter mentored by him? This was not asked directly or indirectly of the whole group, so the sample is quite small. For what it is worth, the respondents answered in the negative.

7. Would he sacrifice his job for a core principle? Most didn't know how to answer this one. Two believed that his close ties to the Bush family and the Bush agenda mean that this issue would probably never come up.

My own experience with Dr. von Eschenbach is limited. Personally, he is affable, sincere, and dedicated to patients with cancer. By all accounts he was a very good urologist when he cared for his patients. I have disagreed with some of his policies, most specifically with his decision to stop funding the National Cancer Policy Board of the Institute of Medicine, which I chaired at the time. His reason was that it didn't have members who were Nobel laureates and because "I don't like committees I can't control." That decision was his right and he did agree to fund another version of that committee, the National Cancer Policy Forum, provided that members of his staff and of other sponsoring government agencies had permanent seats.

Will he be a good leader of the FDA? Some say no because of his lack of research experience and his record at NCI. Personally, I don't know. For all of our sakes, and especially for our current and future patients, I sincerely hope he does well...and does good.

10 May 2006

Reference

[1] Collins JC: Good to great: *Why some companies make the leap ....and others don't.* New York, NY. Harper Collins Publishers, Inc, 2001

LEADERSHIP IN MEDICINE

The Five Deadly Sins of Leadership

THIS ESSAY, THE THIRD IN A SERIES on leadership and management (*see pp 184-189*) describes the condensed wisdom of Peter Drucker, an icon of business management wisdom. It became clear when reading his works that the key values he describes can be applied to leadership in the "cancer industry," from the Food and Drug Administration, the National Cancer Institute (NCI), and pharmaceutical companies to academic medical centers and oncology practices. The "sins" of leadership described below can be seen in the non-profit as well as the for-profit industry, and in professional businesses such as academic departments and private medical practices.

Drucker wrote an article for *The Wall Street Journal* in 1993 entitled, "The Five Deadly Business Sins." It was reprinted in the 21 October 2005 issue of the Journal following Drucker's death.[1] What prompted the article was the downward slide in the few years before of once-dominant businesses such as General Motors (GM), IBM, and Sears. He believed that each was guilty of at least one of five business sins. Some of these come uncomfortably close to describing recognizable "sins" in the oncology world. Keep in mind that Drucker calls these "sins" because they are bad for business, not necessarily for one's soul or moral compass (though Drucker has made the argument that good business practices and high ethical standards are often aligned).

Sin #1: Worship of high profit margins and "premium pricing."
Drucker says this is the most common of the deadly business sins and offers several examples. Xerox invented the copier but kept adding features to increase the profit margin. But most consumers needed a plain copier at reasonable cost; when Canon brought one out it proceeded to dominate the United States market for years. General Motors neglected the market for smaller, more fuel-efficient cars even after the oil crisis of the 1970s, consciously ceding that market to Volkswagen and Japanese car makers. Only after the latter controlled that large market did GM try to respond, but GM remains behind 30 years later because the Japanese cars have been of consistently higher quality.

The pharmaceutical company functions as a legal monopoly with a new drug because of patent protection and will charge "what the market will bear." But is that bad business? Drucker would say yes. Xerox and GM made billions of dollars early in their downward spiral, but the market eventually caught up with them and we see the consequences three decades later. Xerox is now a minor player in copiers and there is talk, only half-jokingly, that Toyota may buy GM.

And we can point to ourselves for what has happened to oncology practices, both academic and community-based. While chemotherapy revenues were soaring, reaching an average of 65% or more of all revenues, there was no agitation to improve the paltry reimbursement for seeing and managing the patient, so practices became dependent on that single source of revenue. The Medicare Modernization Act has severely reduced the profit from the resale of drugs so many patients are being sent to hospitals for their chemotherapy, especially from small practices, which have been the hardest hit. And larger practices are scrambling to reorganize into buying consortiums and to own lucrative diagnostic or radiation therapy facilities to make up for the income "shortfall."

The key difference between the cancer industry on the one hand and Xerox and GM on the other are that patients are not machine products. So the consequences of charging desperate patients tens of thousands of dollars for minimally effective cancer treatment are exponentially greater and, I would argue, more relevant to the cancer industry, not less. There is a strong moral-ethical as well as a business case for addressing these "sins."

Sin #2: Mispricing a new product by charging "what the market will bear."
This is simply an extension of Sin #1. Drucker offers an interesting example of an American company that did it right. DuPont has remained on top of the synthetic fiber industry. When DuPont developed nylon, it priced the patented product at the price they would have to charge in five years to stay competitive. They sacrificed short-term profits for long-term stability and, in the long run, greater profits.

Sin #3: Reliance on cost-driven pricing.
Most companies total up their costs and add a profit to arrive at the sales price. They do this because "we must recover our costs and make a profit." But the market often changes due to competition, government regulation, or unforeseen production or distribution problems. So the company then must cut the price or redesign the product.

Drucker says the alternative and wiser approach is the opposite: "price-driven costing." That is, price a product or service to what the market is willing to pay and control the costs to fit the price. If one takes this approach, the competition will have a hard time undercutting the price and grabbing market share. This would be a hard sell at every level of the cancer industry. Certainly, the NCI finds itself facing serious reductions in research grants because the Congress believes it isn't doing a good job. Whatever the merits of Congress's judgment, the recent large investment in nanotechnology, proteomics, and bioinformatics at the cost of creative research demonstrates either NCI's lack of planning for what "the market will bear" or a misunderstanding of how research progress is and always has been made: by a pool of creative individual investigators that teach the next generation of creative investigators. Each is a potentially fatal error for the future of biomedical research.

Sin #4: Slaughtering tomorrow's opportunity on the altar of yesterday.
IBM brought out the first personal computer (PC), but consciously ceded that new and growing business to Apple and then many others to focus on its lucrative mainframe business. It is said that IBM forbade its PC salesmen to sell to its mainframe customers. It forced the development of PC clones, which businesses wanted. IBM recently sold even its successful laptop business to Lenovo, a Chinese company, and has changed its business model to feature consulting.

The cancer industry (all of us in research, production, and care) is in danger of making the same error. Reliance and continued investment in marginally effective diagnostics and therapies at enormous cost to patients, the public, and to the government keep the industry profitable. But one can argue that this failure by the industry to call into question the true value of these approaches for general use– proton-beam therapy, expensive targeted drugs (when did we ever give drugs we believed were not targeted?) for lung cancer that extend life on average only a few weeks–is the same as IBM sticking with the mainframes.

Sin #5 Feeding problems and starving opportunities.
This is a variant of Sin #4. Drucker illustrates this with an anecdote. He says he always asks new clients who their best-performing people are and where they are assigned. In almost all cases they are assigned to problems—old products, fading lines of business, old technology. He then asks, "Who takes care of opportunities?" Their development is usually left to less able performers who are often left to fend for themselves. He believes Sears has been doing this for years. He said GE on the other hand "gets rid of all old business, even if profitable, that do not offer long-range growth and the opportunity for the company to be number one or two world-wide."

The biomedical research community of the United States, funded largely by the National Institutes of Health, is number one in the world. I would argue it is because its main focus has been its priority of supporting research project grants that are competitively awarded. Although large-scale projects such as nanotechnology, bioinformatics, and proteomics have merit, I question whether the NCI can ever be number one or number two in these areas. It has little strength in technology development. And such expenditures come at the extremely high cost of squeezing many scientists, especially the up-and-comers, out of the business. The result: the pay lines for investigator-initiated grants are shrinking toward single digits.

Peter Drucker's words should give us pause about the direction of the NCI and the whole cancer business. Admittedly, it is difficult to see how individuals can address these issues. It will require an open-minded leadership at NCI to invite an analysis of its portfolio by competent extramural scientists and clinical investigators. If the next director and the Congress continue in the current direction, a decade or two from now the United States will no longer be number one in cancer research and, by extension, biomedical research. Just keep in mind the letters SGX—Sears, GM, and Xerox.

25 May 2006

Reference

[1] Drucker P: The five deadly business sins. *The Wall Street Journal*, October 21, 2005 (reprinted from October 21, 1993)

Pruning the Rosebush

MY GARDENING IS LIMITED BY MY IMPATIENCE and my unwillingness to spend hours crouching or on my knees. Okay, so I'm lazy. But there are some aspects of maintaining plants that I do willingly, almost instinctively. One of these is pruning hybrid tea rose bushes. To have the best blossoms for the longest time, one must have removed dead wood and once blooming begins, one must remove spent blossoms. Both actions take little time and stimulate new growth. One is tempted to leave a blossom that is well past its prime, but retains some color and scent; I have done this many times. But when I do that, I find that I have reduced the bush's productivity and diminished its overall appearance and the pleasure it brings. So I prune without remorse.

Although much more difficult, pruning is just as necessary in organizations. The most common reasons for firing an individual in professional life are 1) a lack of performance or productivity, 2) his/her negative impact on the performance or productivity of colleagues, or 3) a clash of his/her personality or values with the culture of the workplace. Some organizations fire too readily, but the vast majority fire too little or too late, especially in academia and government. Tenure, legal or practical, is often blamed for not firing incompetents, and with good reason (full disclosure: I am opposed to tenure in professional schools).

But more often, the incompetent or destructive individual is left in place because the leader doesn't want the unpleasantness and hassle of removing the individual, the culture of the organization frowns on it, or someone fears a lawsuit. One approach is to try to transfer or hide the individual in hopes that will contain the damage, but that seldom works because a determined malcontent can always find ways to hurt the organization. Even more important is the message sent to all the "good" employees: we won't get rid on an incompetent, so you work harder to make up for his low productivity and put up with his behavior. This is not a morale booster.

For most of us in leadership positions, firing people is the hardest part of the job; there are few who take pleasure in wielding such power. Unlike roses, one is dealing with human beings who have families and responsibilities. Depending on the circumstances, firing a professional will certainly harm his or her career development and, in some extreme cases, may even end it. There are rare circumstances when it is relatively easy to fire a professional, such as cases of fraud, theft, or other major unethical or criminal behavior. But even then, one is left with a feeling of profound sadness.

There are two main types of "firing": firing someone from an "appointed" position or from employment altogether. Appointed positions in academia include dean, chairman of a department, division head, or cancer center director. In those cases, the person may be fired from the appointed job, but retain an often tenured professorship. In community practice it includes medical director at a hospital or an administrative role in the practice itself. Being fired from an appointed position will hurt one's ego, but it doesn't usually threaten one's livelihood. Separating one from the organization is a different matter.

Firing someone from employment may appear to be pretty clear cut for most individuals, but it isn't that easy, especially when dealing with professionals. In academia one must deal with tenure, in private practice with partnerships, and in all types of employment with contracts, grievances, Equal Employment Opportunity Commission issues, etc.

So it is always a good idea to go to great lengths to minimize the likelihood of firing an individual. In addition to the usual screening and obtaining references, I am a believer in screening professional candidates by phone call. I believe the future boss or peer should talk to people from the candidate's current institution(s) or practice(s). This is especially effective if one knows the person called. Written recommendations are often formulaic and not very useful, though a skillfully written letter to an experienced recruiter can implicitly reveal a great deal. People are often much more open on a phone call and will say things or hint at things they would not put in writing. I have been dumbfounded by the frequency of individuals, both high achievers and low, being hired by another organization without any request for recommendations.

But despite all precautions, everyone in a leadership position will surely face the prospect of firing someone. Of course, it should never be done lightly, but when the productivity of the organization is severely or chronically compromised, the individual should be nudged out if possible, or thrown out if necessary. That is a leader's responsibility—to get best available people and to create an environment conducive to fulfilling their potential and the organization's.

There is a circumstance that requires a different approach; I call it the "bad fit." In my experience, this has been the most common situation I faced. An employee may work hard, have good values, and get along with colleagues but is not right for the organization. The organization's culture may have well-established expectations beyond the capability of the individual no matter how hard he works; a smart, hard-working individual who everybody likes who just can't cut it. His or her work lacks something, such as imagination or sufficient detail in their research, always being a step behind clinically, or an inability to write up work. Whatever it is, it is just a bad fit for that environment.

For a bad fit, the solution is to help them find a more suitable environment. Be very clear that they must go, but give them time to find another position, coach them on where to look, make some calls for them. They may not thank you for any help you provide...after all, you are firing them. But you will be able to sleep better and you can provide an honest reference, e.g., "he works hard, but the chemistry here just didn't work out—it is my fault as much as his."

Pruning a rose bush is necessary for the greatest achievement of its beauty and productivity. Firing a person occasionally—one hopes rarely—is necessary for the health and productivity of an organization. It should be a last resort after every attempt has been made to save the situation, but when all else fails it becomes the sad duty of the leader, for the good of all in the organization.

25 August 2006

LEADERSHIP IN MEDICINE

Understanding Effective Leadership

TRYING TO UNDERSTAND LEADERSHIP, good and bad, has been an endlessly fascinating journey for me. And I am not alone. The shelves in the business section at Barnes and Noble are filled with books on the subject and airport concessions, even in smaller airports, always have such books. The *Harvard Business Review* reliably prints many articles, universities offer continuing education courses, and celebrities give well-paid lectures on leadership. Why is the subject so popular? The answer is easy: because leadership is difficult and because leadership is so important to any enterprise.

A parenthetic note of caution here about business books: I have read my share and found the majority to be useless; they are filled with simplistic nostrums, are endlessly repetitive, and have an almost total dependence on anecdotes (case studies), which by their nature are totally retrospective and uncontrolled. Only a small percentage of books provide an enlightening synthesis or novel viewpoints, so *caveat emptor*.

In my own case, an interest in the qualities of effective leaders has been greatly intensified beyond sporadic reading my own experience as a leader of academic programs and hospitals and through my consulting work, which provides opportunities to examine in detail the work and effectiveness of many leaders in health care.

In an earlier essay (*pp 182-184*) I described what some experts believe makes a great leader; or rather, what kind of performance and outcome is apparent in very successful leaders. This is an important distinction. It is much easier to identify an effective leader after the fact than before or during his or her tenure. This raises interesting questions, such as: Are leaders made or born? Can someone be taught to be an effective leader? Can one identify an effective leader beforehand? Are all effective leaders "successful?" I hope to shed a bit of light on these issues from the literature and personal experience.

Are leaders born?

Yes, partly. I agree with Bill George, a former corporate chief executive officer and currently a trustee of large corporations. In his book, *True North: Discover Your Authentic Leadership*, he expresses in several ways that the core characteristics of leadership, the soul of leadership, cannot be taught.1 I have come to believe that what is true for most skillful activities is also true for leadership. Not only is one's DNA a major influence, but George points out that personal crises and other life experiences early in life and later also prepare one to be an effective leader.

Although I loved the game, no matter how hard I tried, I could never have been a competitive college football player. I was the wrong size and shape, terribly slow, and had other interests that were more important to me. A friend once told me of a conversation he had with a chief executive officer of a large corporation. He asked the CEO how he could tell if a candidate was likely to be an effective leader. He replied, "Simple, I just asked them what they did in high school." He was making a point that the signs of an aptitude for leadership show up early.

Can one teach effective leadership?
Only partly and only if the basic soul of leadership is already there, I believe. One can be taught certain techniques and skills through mentoring and graduated experience. But that is a refinement of the basic foundation of good instincts about human nature, character, ambition, and self-confidence. I also believe one can teach, or try to teach, a potential leader that unless he/she gets pleasure out of seeing those being led succeed and get the glory because of his/her efforts, a leadership position may not be a good choice, no matter what other talents are in place.

Can one identify an effective leader beforehand?
This is difficult and typical search processes often fail to identify the right leader for the specific job. In my view, the best predictor of an effective leader is evidence of effective leadership in the past. This seems to be a Catch 22: "I don't know if you will be an effective leader unless you have already been an effective leader. How can one become an effective leader if one never gets the chance?" But this is not as dumb as it sounds. If someone has had experience as a leader, even in a voluntary or relatively minor position, it usually means that the person wanted to be a leader and went after the job, or was recognized by others as someone they would like as their leader. If he/she were successful in that role, that provides a degree of greater security in the evaluation.

In my personal experience, there are two top reasons for the failure of leaders. First, a candidate is hired for the wrong reasons, e.g. an outstanding scientist is hired to be chairman of a department or a dean primarily because of a long bibliography and an expansive curriculum vitae. These are poor indicators of an aptitude for leadership, yet are often the most powerful influence on the decision to hire. Second, the candidate likes the position for its stature and power, but doesn't really like (or understand) the job of leadership. This type often is just a boss or even a bully, but not an effective leader that leads the team to perform at its best.

Are all effective leaders successful?
No. This is one of the great faults of business books on leadership. Too often the only measure of an effective corporate leader is an increase in market share or stock price. In academia, it is grants obtained or papers published. Books don't sell if they describe the leader who, despite seemingly insurmountable obstacles, managed to bring his so-so team to a much higher level of performance than expected. Or the leader who inherited a staff ill-fitted for the job, but was able to rearrange the workforce and work flow to help them perform at their very best. The athletic directors of college sports know this well. They often hire a coach who has turned a chronically losing team at a second or third tier sports college into one that wins half its games. They recognize the coaching talent despite the mediocre player talent.

In summary, effective leaders are born with an innate aptitude that is shaped and grown by life experiences and refined by mentorship and experience; all three are necessary. Although not fail-safe, one makes a better bet on a prospective leader who has a record of successful leadership in the past, no matter at what level. Finally, excellent and effective leaders may not be judged successful by the world's standards, but they may have done an excellent job with the resources and conditions provided—and they usually know that in their hearts.

25 May 2007

Reference
[1] George B, Sims P, Gergen D. *True North: Discover Your Authentic Leadership.* San Francisco, CA. Jossey-Bass, 2007

Chapter 7

CANCER RESEARCH

I have been involved in cancer research in one way or another for my entire career. Research is a mixture of courage, hard work, and a great deal of trial and error, with a dash of inspiration. I include essays here that provide a flavor of the issues medical researchers face every day, and I describe some successes and failures of the "system" created for such research.

CANCER RESEARCH

Childhood Cancer Research: A Victim of Success and Bureaucracy

ONE COULD ARGUE CONVINCINGLY that pediatric oncology, my own subspecialty, has been the most successful force of modern oncology in treatment successes, lives saved, and clinical research productivity. At least three-quarters of all children treated for cancer in the last decade are long-term survivors and nearly that many are cured of cancer.

How did this happen? The main reason is biology. Pediatric tumors predominantly arise from embryonic tissue and are inherently more sensitive to current therapy. Adult tumors are overwhelmingly carcinomas that arise from epithelial tissue, and most are relatively insensitive to current therapy. But there has been another contributing factor.

The system of care for children with cancer differs significantly from the care for adults with cancer. Most children are treated at childhood cancer centers, all of which participate in clinical trials. Consequently, a large fraction, perhaps 50% or more, of all children with cancer are treated according to a peer-reviewed protocol. Although many of the protocols consist of empirical variations of those from prior studies rather than dramatically novel therapies, this mix of approaches has proved effective. An example is childhood acute lymphoblastic leukemia. The cure rate has increased progressively from about 10-15% in the mid-1970s to nearly 80% today, despite the lack of any new mainline chemotherapy agents in that time. At the same time, childhood acute lymphoblastic leukemia has been a hotbed of immunologic, cytogenetic, and molecular innovation.

Perhaps an even greater effect of the widespread use of protocols has been that standards for pathology, surgery, imaging, radiation therapy, and chemotherapy were established in these institutions and soon were applied to patients whether or not they were treated according to a protocol, thus weaving a fine cultural fabric of research and care. This engendered an atmosphere of high standards, cooperation, and enthusiastic participation. However, there are worrisome signs that the fabric of that culture is fraying.

First, we are victims of our own success. As overall cure rates approach or exceed 75% in some cancers, launching radical innovations is more difficult for fear of endangering sure cures. But substantive innovation not only drives research, it powers enthusiasm and optimism and attracts top trainees interested in research. Caution is warranted; reticence is not.

Second is the troubled merger of the Pediatric Oncology Group (POG) and the Children's Cancer Group (CCG) to form the Children's Oncology Group (COG). To date, the COG has made little if any progress in attaining the primary objectives of the merger, i.e., greater efficiency and productivity, lower cost, and more patients on trials. Furthermore, the spirit of optimism and cooperation certainly has suffered. Some former CCG and POG members have complained that the COG structure allows fewer opportunities for leading studies and suffers from a painfully slow process for getting protocols designed and approved. These bureaucratic problems may fade with time, but meanwhile another movement is gaining steam.

Groups of five or more pediatric institutions have been forming research consortia for the study of neuroblastoma, brain tumors, Hodgkin's disease, acute myeloid leukemia, and others. With the smaller membership, meetings can be more intimate, agreement quicker, meaningful participation virtually assured, and the opportunity for innovation greater. The larger the committee, the less likely it will innovate.

Is this a good time for a new strategic model, such as a federation of smaller groups of institutions, for this changed environment? For example, two or three neuroblastoma groups might be better because they would generate independent research vectors and would also have the virtue of a built-in peer-review system for collaborative competition. The COG as a whole would continue to focus on large-scale phase 3 studies. An open discussion would certainly generate other models to consider.

Pediatric oncology has been the innovator for many facets of oncology. Its institutional and cooperative group leaders have an opportunity to reconsider and debate its direction and structure to ensure its leadership role in the future. It would be a tragedy if pediatric oncology were to decline as a vibrant, innovative scientific craft because of insufficient attention to strategic and organizational issues.

25 September 2003

CANCER RESEARCH

Childhood Cancer: An Orphan of New Drug Development

PEDIATRIC ONCOLOGY HAS ARGUABLY BEEN the most successful force of modern oncology in treatment successes, lives saved and clinical research productivity. At least three-quarters of all children treated for cancer in the last decade are long-term survivors and nearly that many are cured of cancer. The biology of childhood cancers makes many of them more sensitive to therapy, but the system of care for children with cancer and the large participation in clinical trials contributes to this success.

However, about 25% of children are not cured, and the intensive multi-agent therapy responsible for this success has levied significant costs in acute and long-term side effects. Scientific progress in the past decade has not led to substantial improvements in survival or cure. One reason is that few new agents have been developed specifically for childhood cancer; the last front-line agent for the most common childhood cancer, acute lymphoblastic leukemia, was introduced 30 years ago. Therein lies the rub.

Because childhood cancer is relatively rare, pharmaceutical companies tell us that developing drugs specific for its treatment is not economically viable; the market is too small to justify the enormous expense. The problem is the same as for rare "orphan" diseases with a few hundred to a few thousand cases per year. This is a serious threat to progress in pediatric oncology (see the editorial by Robert Wittes in *The New England Journal of Medicine*[1]).

I have asked Peter Adamson to help us understand the problem and what is and should be done about it. Dr. Adamson is a pediatric oncologist and clinical pharmacologist at the Children's Hospital of Philadelphia and the University of Pennsylvania and Chair of the Developmental Therapeutics program for the Children's Oncology Group (COG). He is an expert in drug therapy and drug development for childhood cancer. He is an expert in drug therapy and drug development for childhood cancer.

Q: *Wasn't federal legislation passed to solve some of these problems?*
Adamson: There have been two complementary sets of legislation aimed at improving upon the situation in which two-thirds of medications prescribed today lack pediatric

information in their label. Overall, the impact of the 1997 Food and Drug Administration Modernization Act (FDAMA) incentive program, replaced by the Best Pharmaceuticals for Children Act of 2002, has been relatively limited in cancer chemotherapy. FDAMA has had its greatest impact in pediatric disease areas for which "blockbuster" drugs exist in adults, such as hypertension. The impact of the Pediatric Research Equity Act of 2003, which replaced the Pediatric Final Rule, is not yet known. If drugs continue to be labeled by pathologic indication only (e.g., prostate cancer), the impact will likely be limited. If drugs become labeled based on molecular target, the act may have a more significant impact for drugs in the development pipeline. For example, a pediatric tumor that relies for its growth on a similar molecular pathway as a common adult cancer would automatically be included in the indications.

Q: *Wasn't part of the legislation crafted to provide an incentive to industry in the form of an extension to exclusivity?*
Adamson: Indeed that is where legislation has had its greatest impact, but the true value of a 6-month extension of exclusivity may not be realized until relatively late in the lifecycle of a drug; thus, there is less incentive for companies to embark on pediatric research for drugs early in clinical development.

Q: *With more than 400 new anticancer agents in the development pipeline, what strategies are you taking for selecting new agents for phase 1 studies in children?*
Adamson: Despite this explosion of new agents, there is still a relative paucity of new agents entering phase 1 trials for children with cancer. Therefore, we are not yet limited by the number of potentially eligible patients in deciding how many studies to open up; in fact, the COG Developmental Therapeutics consortium has increased its efficiency to the extent that we have had to use a waiting list system to enter eligible patients onto studies. An equally important need for us is access to new agents for preclinical testing in childhood cancer models. Industry does not develop nor screen drugs for activity against childhood cancers, so our knowledge of the potential role of agents in the development pipeline for childhood cancer is often quite limited by the time we are ready to embark on clinical studies.

Q: *In that case, what is being done to address preclinical testing for childhood cancer?*
Adamson: Fortunately, language in enacted legislation has directed some federal resources to help address the current situation. The COG Developmental Therapeutics program has responded to the initiative put forward by the NCI to begin to systematically test new agents in the clinical development pipeline in a series of pediatric cancer models. Peter Houghton from St. Jude is leading this effort on our behalf. He has assembled a pre-clinical consortium of academic investigators who are well positioned to work

with industry sponsors and the NCI in systematically evaluating a panel of pediatric preclinical models that will help prioritize new agents for study in children with cancer.

Q: *What are the clinical research challenges that lay ahead in this arena?*
Adamson: Phase 1 is relatively straightforward, although many of the newer biological agents may not have a traditional "maximum-tolerated dose." The real challenge in children will be phase 2 studies, as many of these new agents will need to be delivered in combination with cytotoxic agents. In pediatrics, we will not have the option to run multiple phase 3 trials to answer combination questions; we will need novel designs beyond standard phase 2 designs. Developing new agents for childhood acute leukemias may be a significant challenge. Historically, such patients were only considered for investigational new drug therapy late in the course of refractory disease, and accrual has been difficult. New design paradigms are being explored.

Q: *What about developing agents specifically aimed at molecular targets unique to childhood cancer?*
Adamson: This will prove to be our ultimate challenge. Academic medicine is good at defining targets, but understanding the functional significance of targets is as much of a challenge in childhood cancer as in adult cancer. Industry is not going to take the lead here, but we do need its expertise and a collaborative access to molecular libraries once we have identified a target and validated an assay to screen for drugs.

Q: *Since developing new drugs for childhood cancer is not financially sustainable for industry, are there alternative ways to do this?*
Adamson: We will need to think outside the box to begin to address this challenge. One proposal being discussed by a number of experts is developing a public-private partnership to address this. We know that many of the components needed to develop new drugs for childhood cancers already exist but are not yet being utilized for this purpose. Universities, academic medical centers, the pharmaceutical industry, and the NCI must partner in this endeavor. What is needed is a mechanism to drive the process and allow the relevant parties to contribute their expertise and research capacities at the appropriate points in the process. An Institute of Medicine subcommittee is examining the potential for such an approach, and will hopefully set the framework for developing a system that has the capability to develop targeted therapies unique to childhood cancers. That report should be completed by the end of the year.

25 June 2004

Reference
[1] Wittes R: Therapy for cancer in children—Past successes, future challenges. *N Engl Jrl Med* 348:747-749, 2003

CANCER RESEARCH

NCI Cancer Centers Program – A Jewel Needing Polish

CANCER CENTERS THAT ARE PEER REVIEWED and supported by the National Cancer Institute ("NCI centers") have been an integral part of the cancer research enterprise in this country for over three decades. In many ways, the program has been one of the great success stories among National Institutes of Health extramural programs. However, the program is showing its age and is a little ragged around the edges. It is not clear whether this is due to problems intrinsic to cancer centers themselves or to extrinsic factors. I will address that question, but the program needs an overhaul if its highest expectations are to be fulfilled.

Before exploring this question, a brief review of the cancer centers program's purpose and features is helpful. The program was established in its current form around 1970 to provide infrastructure for cancer research in academic institutions, to encourage cancer research by more scientists, and to provide a focus for cancer activities in institutions not devoted entirely to cancer. More details are available in overviews of the program.[1,2]

An institution qualifies for a Cancer Center Support Grant in two primary ways: 1) to the degree to which it has funded high-quality research in actively coordinated cancer programs; and 2) how well it fulfills the six essential characteristics of a center, i.e., institutional commitment, cancer focus, qualifications and authority of the director, organizational capability, facilities, and interdisciplinary and transdisciplinary collaboration and coordination. These characteristics are by far the most important of the qualifying requirements.

Let's consider an assessment of the cancer centers program as a whole. The program has been highly successful in fulfilling its first initial goal. It has provided important and sometimes critical infrastructure for cancer research. It has allowed the development of shared resources for essential and sometimes innovative technology. The grants have provided resources for research development, recruitment of new faculty, and seed funding for young investigators and for established investigators venturing into new territory. The grants have also provided for essential administrative support and have allowed modest payment to key leaders to cover a portion of their time.

The program has also been successful in its second main goal, attracting scientists into cancer research who would not otherwise have done so. Preferred access to shared facilities run by the cancer center and an opportunity to play a role in research organized around a single disease are two of several reasons.

The program has been most successful, in my view, in its third main goal: providing a focus for cancer activities in institutions not devoted entirely to cancer. While categorical cancer institutions such as MD Anderson, Memorial Sloan-Kettering, and Fox Chase would focus on cancer research and patient care with or without an NCI centers program, the majority of NCI centers are in medical schools and universities in which cancer is only one of many areas of interest and activity. It is in these settings that the program has had its greatest impact. Many of these "matrix" centers have taken advantage of the diversity of expertise found in medical schools and universities to greatly enrich the cancer research activities to a degree impossible without the cancer center. In many cases, the cancer center has become a unifying force on campuses and a major source of revenue from grants, philanthropy, and clinical activity.

These successes have led to periodic flashes of great cancer research. In addition, centers have often become a barometer of excellence, leadership and innovation for the medical and public communities in their regions. It is not a stretch to say, therefore, that after research project grants, the cancer centers program has been the most important, effective, and productive effort of the NCI.

But all is not well in the cancer centers program. According to a broad sample of opinions from senior leaders in many NCI centers, there is substantial room for improvement and the recent budget woes have put many of the concerns in sharp relief. One might consider such complaints self-serving, but because of the long history of the centers' success and my personal experience with the productivity of the centers, I am inclined to believe that the problems are not intrinsic to the cancer centers themselves. Here is a summary of several of the areas of concern that leaders have expressed.

First, the review process has become unnecessarily complex, numbingly formulaic, and incredibly burdensome, often requiring several person-years to prepare for each competitive renewal. The process does not assess the quality of research in sufficient depth and spends too much time on numerical information such as financial status, research grant dollars, and number of patients and minorities on clinical trials, so everyone is counting beans. An excessive focus on administrative processes eventually diminishes the importance of science in the review and leads to a greater emphasis on grantsmanship, bookkeeping, and theatrics. Eventually, the process can reward scientific mediocrity disguised by the Potemkin village façade of rigorous bean counting. This arcane review process sometimes results in the appearance of unfairness in the priority score. This counting is necessary and important but not at the expense of a thorough scientific review.

Second, there has been a steady erosion of flexibility allowed to the centers. It is now widely held that the review process has progressively constricted the degrees of freedom and is pressing all centers to look and behave alike. The fact that each center has unique strengths and resides in a unique scientific and clinical environment is often dismissed as irrelevant. But the ability of each center to focus and excel in particular areas has been one of the great advantages of the program. A center's particular array of shared resources may justifiably differ from another center, but some are penalized because of a reviewer's personal preference. Another aspect of this constriction is the attitude that research grants from the NCI are the best, and some believe the only, measure of acceptable cancer research. Using the number of NCI grants as a parameter for funding the Cancer Center Support Grant has subtly reinforced that trend. Clearly, outstanding basic research essential for understanding cancer is funded by other institutes and foundations.

Third, there is a strong feeling that the current budgetary situation could at least have been mitigated, if not avoided, since the problem was foreseen even before the doubling of the NCI budget was completed near the end of the Klausner era. There apparently was no plan to try for a soft landing. Instead, the paylines are now dangerously narrow, existing grants are being cut, and programs are being scaled back. This problem is not limited to Cancer Center Support Grants, of course. Individual research project grants have also been squeezed, with young investigators suffering the most. It is these grants that are the heart of the cancer center and by which the center is judged worthy to receive a Cancer Center Support Grant. There is a feeling that either someone was asleep at the switch at the NCI or the funding priorities were upside down, or both.

If my view is correct that the cancer centers program is the single most potent engine of cancer research of the NCI, then what could be done to make it better? I offer three ideas; cancer center leaders and NCI staff will certainly have others.

My first idea is that the review process should focus much more on the quality and innovation of research. The second major focus of the review should be on how well the institution meets the essential characteristics of NCI centers. The scientific review should be made more substantive (research programs often are given only 10 minutes for presentations at site visits) and not diluted by bean counting. This accounting part could be tabulated separately by NCI staffers and peer reviewed separately by cancer center administrators and other leaders; thus, the review by scientists could focus mainly on scientific issues. This change would also allow time for scientists to assess the value of the cancer research supported by agencies other than NCI instead of taking the unjust shortcut of assessing research value by the source of funds.

To emphasize the importance of the science and the six essential characteristics, the priority score could be weighted primarily on those issues. For example, scientific excellence and innovation (in the collaborative context of a cancer center) might count for

50% of the priority score; meeting essential characteristics, 35%; and all the rest, could count for 15%. Or it might be 50-30-20. In either case, research excellence would count for half and cancer center qualities for half. In my view, this would make preparation of the grant less onerous, the review process more relevant, and the priority score more understandable.

Let me be clear; the NCI has an obligation to assess how the money is spent, and the above recommendation is not meant to disparage or minimize that responsibility. However, the review process can and should be handled in such a way that scientists spend the bulk of their time reviewing science in more detail.

My second idea is that the diversity of cancer centers should be encouraged and basic science grants from other institutes that fund excellent research on basic cellular and molecular mechanisms should be given the same value as NCI grants. Who knows where advances will come from? As long as the science is strong and the center functions as such, unique approaches should be permitted, even encouraged.

My third idea is that input from representatives of the cancer centers should be obtained early in the process of dealing with severe budget shortfalls and setting priorities. It is the prerogative and responsibility of the NCI leaders to make budgetary decisions, but in such difficult times it is wise to have the people who actually do the research engaged, well-informed, and inside the tent.

Cancer centers are the jewels of the NCI's extramural program; jewels need periodic buffing to fully express their brilliance.

25 July 2006

References

[1] The National Cancer Institute Cancer Centers Program
http://www.cancer.gov/cancertopics/factsheet/NCI/cancer-centers

[2] Simone JV: Understanding cancer centers. *J Clin Oncol* 20:4503-4507, 2002

CANCER RESEARCH

The Transformation of Cancer Research

WE CLINICIANS, ESPECIALLY THOSE OF US some decades removed from our formal training, often have a difficult time understanding advances in basic cancer research. The jargon used in basic research is continually changing and it sounds like a foreign language (basic scientists say the same about clinical presentations). It requires a sustained effort on my part to maintain at least a nodding acquaintance with the language and movement of basic cancer research. I do it out of curiosity and because I think it is an important means of evaluating new therapies. Major sources of this information are symposia at annual medical meetings. I make a point of listening to at least two or three basic science presentations; I seem to absorb the information better at such sessions than by reading journals because the context and visuals are usually richer and the message clearer.

At the recent joint meeting of the Association of American Physicians and the American Society for Clinical Investigation in Chicago, I heard a talk by Dr. Harold Varmus that was emblematic of the remarkable transformation of cancer research over the past decade or so. Varmus is the president of Memorial Sloan-Kettering Cancer Center (MSKCC), the former director of the National Institutes of Health (NIH) and a Nobel Laureate for his work on the genetics of carcinogenesis.

He also is representative of the MD-scientist whose work has been based entirely in the laboratory. Over many years of medical administration, scientists like Dr. Varmus and the PhDs who are virtually indistinguishable, had little or no interest in clinical oncology. Few made even a meager effort to understand our problems and progress, or lack thereof. And clinicians rarely attended basic-science seminars. This gulf seemed permanent.

How things have changed! Dr. Varmus's talk included chest films of a patient before and after the administration of an experimental therapeutic agent. When he showed the customary list of those who actually did the work he described, it included full-time surgeons and medical oncologists. He pointed out that the lung cancer group at MSKCC that includes clinicians and scientists met every Monday morning at 8:00am to discuss ongoing and future research experiments. This is not an isolated incident—such meetings are now held in many cancer centers—but for an old-timer like me, it is a revolutionary change.

What brought on this change? In my opinion, the single most important factor has been the progressive convergence of the interests of basic and clinical scientists driven by the introduction of new technologies. Dr. Sidney Brenner, a Nobel Laureate is quoted as stating, "Progress in science depends on new technologies, new discoveries and new ideas, probably in that order." Contemporary cancer genetics, with its emerging reliance on genomic approaches, revealed that the genetic diversity within specific types of human cancers was much wider than had been previously appreciated. With small groups of patients exhibiting variant genetic profiles, their study required a large number of tissue samples, and in particular, well-annotated samples, i.e., with fairly detailed clinical information.

The days of scientists simply saying "send me some breast cancer tissue" were gone; with the increasing genetic subclassifications of cancer, the tissue alone was no longer sufficient for this kind of study and the clinicians no longer were simply a source of tissue, but a source of valuable and essential clinical information and its interpretation.

A second factor accelerated the change: the study and development of imatinib (Gleevec) by Brian Druker and Charles Sawyers with two scientists at Novartis, Nick Lyton and Alex Matter. It was a bombshell in the cancer research community, even more so among basic scientists. It provided clear proof-of-principle that a small molecule that targeted the founding genetic lesion in a particular cancer could shrink the cancer and induce durable remissions with few or no side effects.

In his talk, Varmus covered three areas: 1) a description of what he called the "Big Ideas" of cancer research from 1970 to the present; 2) a description of the work of the lung cancer group at MSKCC with gefitinib (Iressa) and other agents; and 3) some new approaches to the development of anticancer agents. I will summarize a few of his points.

The "Big Ideas" in cancer research since 1970, in roughly chronological order were as follows. 1) Cancer-causing genes are mutated versions of oncogenes and tumor suppressor genes. 2) Protein products of the mutant genes have varied functions, e.g., enzymes or transcription factors. 3) Cancer genes *maintain* as well as initiate cancer (remember the "maintain" part in particular). And for me the newest and most interesting was 4) Cancer cells may become "addicted" to the oncogenic proteins and require those products for their continued survival.

Varmus also discussed some clinical studies of patients with lung cancer. As most readers know, patients given gefitinib were most likely to respond positively if they had a mutation of an epidermal growth factor (EFG) receptor. And resistance eventually developed in the responders, often due to secondary mutations that bypass EGF receptor signaling. In this regard, the studies of drug resistance in chronic myelocytic leukemia are much better documented. Leukemias that fail to respond to imatinib therapy almost always return with a mutation in the BCR-ABL kinase that confers drug resistance. The newest drug now in phase 3 studies, dasatinib, "hits" most mutant forms of BCR-ABL and is proving to be a more potent clinical agent as a result.

Finally, Varmus listed what he believed to be the most important avenues of cancer research: the acquired dependence on its oncoprotein products of the cancer cells; the hierarchy of importance and power of oncogene mutations and tumor suppressor inactivation; the search for new anticancer agents aimed at these new targets; an understanding of the mechanisms of drug resistance to imatinib, gefitinib, and other new agents; and the determination of whether there is such a thing as cancer stem cells and, if so, what strategies could be used to eliminate them.

He ended with comments on the necessity of working within the context of cancer research, e.g., a flat NIH budget and the cultural norms of basic and clinical research. He also said the leadership of the NCI must be settled as soon as possible so that appropriate plans can be made and actions taken.

As you might guess from my comments, I thought the talk was very good and demonstrated the clear and sensible leadership that a scientist of Varmus's stature can provide. I wonder: would he be willing to take a huge pay cut to become director of the NCI?

10 June 2006

CANCER RESEARCH

A Cautionary Tale

THE OUTLINES OF THIS STORY are known to most of us, even to me, a pediatric oncologist. In the 1980s, phase 2 studies showed that high-dose chemotherapy followed by autologous bone marrow transplantation was a promising approach for treating metastatic breast cancer. The procedure became so popular that by the 1990s it became accepted by many as the "standard of care." Doctors, hospitals, patients, legislators, patient advocates and, finally, the courts forced insurers to pay for the expensive procedure they had maintained was still experimental.

This wave of acceptance made it difficult to get patients to join randomized controlled trials. When the latter were finally completed and reported at the now-famous plenary session of ASCO in 1999, they showed no therapeutic advantage for the procedure when compared with chemotherapy alone; it also caused much more toxicity. However, there were two randomized trials reported by Dr. Werner Bezwoda of South Africa that showed a significant advantage for the procedure.[1,2] The 1995 study had been criticized for using an atypical control group. Because these were now the only positive randomized studies, they eventually were audited in 2000 by Dr. Raymond Weiss. He and his team found that the data from Bezwoda's studies were fabricated and fraudulent.[3]

The academic and financial structures built around the use of the procedure for adult solid tumors, which had developed over two decades, rapidly collapsed.

False Hope: Bone Marrow Transplantation for Breast Cancer is a new book by Richard Rettig, Peter Jacobson, Cynthia Farquhar, and Wade Aubry, all distinguished health policy scholars.[4] The book addresses one main question: How did this happen? They develop a detailed and well-documented chronology of the events, organizations, people, and health-care financial environment that influenced the course of the story.

The story is not only fascinating, like a complex mystery novel, but many of the players in academia, industry, and private practice are well known to most of us. Although we know how it ends, the specific roles of each person, the critical sequence of events, and the societal changes underway at the time—advocacy, women's rights, managed care, the "more is better" movement in chemotherapy, media portrayal of patients as victims, legislative and judicial activism – provide an intriguing, quilted story. Most of all, it is a cautionary tale for all of us who deal with patients with cancer...or any serious illness.

In this space, I can report only a small sample of the book, so I chose a few examples from those parts I had underlined during my reading. What kept pulling me along in the book was the sequence of events, much of which I had not known. Sadly, there were many opportunities to control the process before it became, with each passing year, a steamroller of inevitability. Ultimately, it became a perfect storm of aligned forces and interests; it was then too late to control it. It finally was stopped, like the perfect storm, only when the energy was dissipated, in this case by the results of the controlled trials.

The main thrust of the story started at the Dana-Farber Cancer Institute in the early 1980s. Key players there at the time under the tutelage of Dr. Emil Frei, a giant in the history of oncology, included Drs. William Peters, Karen Antman, and Craig Henderson, all of whom continued to play major roles until, and beyond, the crash in 1999.

In the 1980s, the prevailing view was, to oversimplify, "more is better." In other words, the reason cancer failed to melt away after chemotherapy was because not enough was given. Either doctors were arbitrarily reducing doses below effective levels or the tumors were resistant to conventional doses. So, a whole series of aggressive, toxic therapies appeared and became fashionable. Since the treatment doses and schedules were so toxic, growth factors became an almost routine part of many regimens in an attempt to mitigate the depression of blood cells and the consequent risk of fatal infection. Thus, the use of high-dose chemotherapy with autologous marrow transplantation was a natural extension of that approach.

The insurance environment at the time played a major role. Managed care was at it apogee; its policies had caused a gradually rising wave of anger among physicians and patients for the denial of payment for expensive treatments, particularly for potentially fatal illnesses. Managed care became the bad guy when it denied coverage of autologous bone marrow transplantation and eventually stood alone against enormous pressure. Bad publicity and, in a few well-publicized cases, the courts eventually caused most insurers to relent.

The book points to an influential 1990 "white paper," apparently never published, that was widely circulated at a crucial moment and helped defeat the insurers. It was titled, "High dose chemotherapy and autologous bone marrow support for breast cancer: a technology assessment." Its authors were Drs. William Peters, Marc Lippman, Gianni Bonadonna, Vincent De Vita, James Holland, and G.L. Rosner. The authors were called a "dream team" by a plaintiff's lawyer. By this time, the procedure was being used not only in stage IV breast cancer, but in stages II and III involving large numbers of axillary nodes. Based on a review of many phase 2 studies, the paper states, "The use of high dose chemotherapy and autologous bone marrow support for selected patients with breast cancer should no longer be considered investigational." And it later states that the evidence favors the procedure over conventional therapy for stages II and III breast cancer involving large numbers of axillary nodes. These were and are distinguished clinical investigators. Their word carried enormous weight and, along with that of many other oncology experts, legitimized the experimental procedure.

The book does a good job of focusing on the most important underlying factor in the story: a conflict of values. The consistent conflict that runs through the whole story was "the need to balance the evaluation of the procedure's effectiveness against making it available to patients before such evidence was firmly established." Does this sound familiar? Oncologists face this conflict of values often and under many circumstances. The most common example is the widespread practice of off-label use of drugs without scientific evidence of effectiveness or, at times, even potential effectiveness. The most forceful driver of this practice is the pressure to "do something, anything" for a desperate patient. That is very hard for us physicians to resist, so an often convoluted rationale is constructed to give the untested treatment.

The authors of the book offer a solution to this problem. Keep in mind that high-dose chemotherapy with autologous bone marrow support is not a drug, but a procedure, so the Food and Drug Administration has no jurisdiction. In fact, there is no agency that has oversight of procedures. The authors therefore propose that a public-private entity under the aegis of the NCI be established to vet such procedures. It sounds good, but such novel procedures are uncommon in oncology and it may be difficult to justify another oversight committee.

Furthermore, there were opportunities to prevent the steamroller from getting out of control. Many counseled greater caution early and often, including Dr. Craig Henderson, Dr. David Eddy, and the Breast Cancer Guidelines Committee of the National Comprehensive Cancer Network. Controlled clinical trials were underway early, but the atmosphere helped prevent earlier completion. Finally, many physicians are ambivalent about controlled clinical trials, and some eminent oncologists, including Drs. Emil Freireich and Samuel Hellman, are dubious of the need or ethical basis for randomized clinical trials.

Although it pains me to say this, we doctors dropped the ball and must take a large share of the responsibility. A visit to the annual ASCO meeting will convince one how desperate we are for any sign, no matter how minor, that a treatment might work for metastatic solid tumors. We share our patients' desperation, but we do them no favor by adopting unproven therapies as the standard of care. It is estimated by Rettig, et al. that from 1998 to 2002, at least 23,000 and as many as 40,000 women received the procedure for breast cancer.[4] There is no requirement that the procedure be reported, so the lower number from the National Inpatient Sample and the American Bone Marrow Transplant Registry is likely a gross underestimate. Setting aside the enormous cost, toxicity from the procedure was often severe, debilitating, and lasting.

Will this happen again? The simultaneous melding of disparate forces coming together as they did, the perfect storm, is likely a rare event. But I venture to guess that something like it will happen again someday because we will always have desperate patients with cancer, doctors susceptible to patients' desperation, a sprinkling of medical entrepreneurs, and the rare fraud. That is to say, human nature won't change. But I highly recommend the book in the hope that through its lessons we can postpone a recurrence for a long time.

10 July 2007

References

[1] Bezwoda WR, Seymour L, Dansey RD: High-dose chemotherapy with hematopoietic rescue as primary treatment for metastatic breast cancer: a randomized trial. *J Clin Oncology* 13:2483-2489, 1995

[2] Plenary session: 1999 American Society of Clinical Oncology Meeting. [http://www.asco.org/portal/site/ASCO/menuitem.64cfbd0f85cb37b2eda2be0aee37a01d/?vgnextoid=09f8201eb61a7010VgnVCM100000ed730ad1RCRD&vmview=vm_session_presentations_view&index=y&confID=17&trackID=2&sessionID=]

[3] Weiss RB, Rifkin RM, Stewart FM, et al: High-dose chemotherapy for high-risk primary breast cancer: An on-site review of the Bezwoda study. *Lancet* 355: 999-1003, 2000

[4] Rettig R, Jacobson P, Farquhar C, Aubry W. *False Hope: Bone Marrow Transplantation for Breast Cancer.* New York, NY. Oxford University Press, 2007

About the Author

DR. JOSEPH V. SIMONE IS PRESIDENT OF SIMONE CONSULTING, clinical director emeritus of the Huntsman Cancer Institute and the professor emeritus of pediatrics and medicine at the University of Utah School of Medicine. He received his medical degree from the Stritch School of Medicine of Loyola University in Chicago in 1960. He completed his training in Chicago with a residency in medicine at Presbyterian-St.Luke's Hospital and a fellowship in pediatric hematology-oncology at the University of Illinois.

Dr. Simone spent most of his medical career at St. Jude Children's Research Hospital in Memphis, where he joined the staff in 1967. In his years there, he was engaged in clinical research efforts to improve therapy for children with cancer; he played a leadership role in the development of curative treatments for childhood leukemia and lymphoma. In 1983, Dr. Simone was named director of St. Jude, at which time he turned his efforts to the administrative leadership of research and the hospital. During Dr. Simone's tenure, St. Jude experienced both a scientific renewal and major growth in its physical facilities.

From 1992 to 1996 he served as physician-in-chief of the Memorial Sloan-Kettering Cancer Center in New York City where he developed several programs aimed at addressing the seismic changes in health care. These included a cancer disease management system and a regional clinical cancer network.

Dr. Simone has served as medical director and chairman of the National Comprehensive Cancer Network and as a member of the Board of Scientific Advisors of the National Cancer Institute (NCI) from 1996 to 2002. He has been a member the National Cancer Policy Board of the Institute of Medicine since 1997 and served as its chairman until 2005. He serves on the external advisory committees of 12 NCI-designated cancer centers. He is past chairman of both the Cancer Clinical Investigators Review Committee and the Cancer Center Review Committee of the National Cancer Institute. He is a former president of the Association of American Cancer Institutes and former vice chairman of the Pediatric Oncology Group.

Among his awards and honors, Dr. Simone was elected to the Association of American Physicians. The American Association for Cancer Research awarded him the Richard and Hinda Rosenthal Foundation Award and the American Society of Clinical Oncology awarded him the Distinguished Service Award for Scientific Excellence in 2002 and the Public Service Award in 2006.

Further information about Dr. Simone is available at www.simoneconsulting.com; he can be contacted via email at simone_j@bellsouth.net.